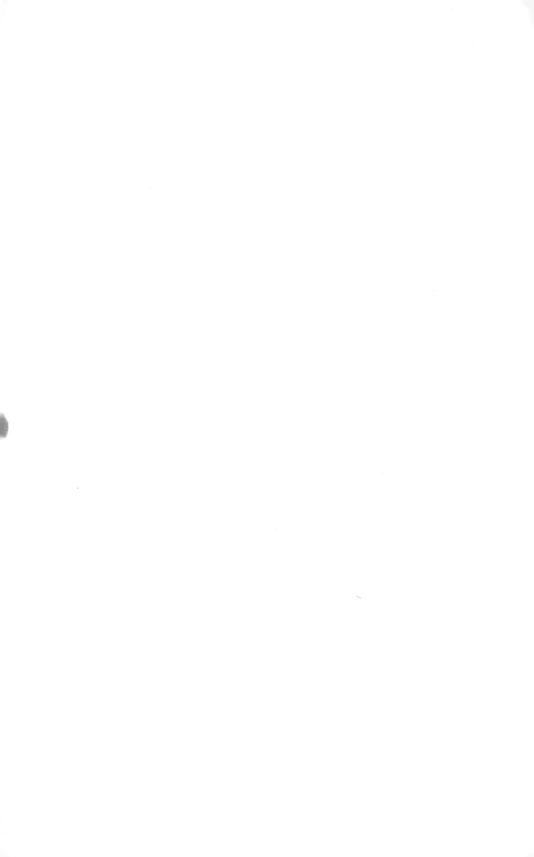

Cholestatic Liver Disease

CLINICAL GASTROENTEROLOGY ™

George Y. Wu, MD, PhD, SERIES EDITOR

CLINICAL GASTROENTEROLOGY™

Cholestatic Liver Disease

Edited by

Keith D. Lindor, MD

Mayo Clinic, Rochester, MN

and

Jayant A. Talwalkar, MD

Mayo Clinic, Rochester, MN

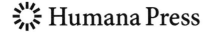 Humana Press

© 2008 Humana Press
999 Riverview Drive, Suite 208
Totowa, New Jersey 07512
www.humanapress.com

This publication is printed on acid-free paper. ∞

ANSI Z39.48-1984 (American National Standards Institute) Permanence of Paper for Printed Library Materials.

Cover illustration: Figure 1, Chapter 4, "Primary Sclerosing Cholangitis," by Kelly Warren Burak, and Figures 1–3, Chapter 5, "Overlap Syndrome with Autoimmune Hepatitis," by Alastair Smith.

Cover design by Karen Schulz

Production Editor: Michele Seugling

For additional copies, pricing for bulk purchases, and/or information about other Humana titles, contact Humana at the above address or at any of the following numbers: Tel: 973-256-1699; Fax: 973-256-8341; or visit our website at http://humanapress.com

Printed in the United States of America.   10 9 8 7 6 5 4 3 2 1
e-ISBN: 978-1-59745-118-5

Library of Congress Control Number: 2007942038

Preface

Over the past two decades, there has been a steady increase in the fund of knowledge associated with the clinical manifestations of cholestatic liver disease. In addition to a growing amount of information on the well-studied disorders of primary biliary cirrhosis and primary sclerosing cholangitis, there has also been a rapid accumulation of data on less well-known but important topics such as overlap syndromes with autoimmune hepatitis, cholestatic variants of alcohol and viral disease, and cholestasis following liver transplantation. In turn, these emerging insights are being complemented by further improvements regarding the diagnosis and management of cholestasis.

Based on these clinical situations, we hope that *Cholestatic Liver Disease* will provide useful information for individuals who are involved in the care of patients affected by various aspects of cholestatic liver disease. The goal of this textbook is to provide scientific updates from leading experts, which relate to the clinical evaluation and management of cholestatic liver disorders. It is our hope that *Cholestatic Liver Disease* will be a useful reference for both learners and practitioners alike.

Keith D. Lindor, MD
Jayant A. Talwalkar, MD

Contents

Contributors

KELLY WARREN BURAK, MD • *University of Calgary Liver Unit, Calgary, Alberta, Canada*

VIRGINIA C. CLARK, MD • *University of Florida, Gainesville, FL*

JEFFREY S. CRIPPIN, MD • *Washington University School of Medicine, St. Louis, MO*

KIMBERLY FORDE, MD • *University of Pennsylvania, Philadelphia, PA*

JAMES P. HAMILTON, MD • *University of Maryland, School of Medicine, Baltimore, MD*

DAVID E. KAPLAN, MD • *University of Pennsylvania, Philadelphia, PA*

SAKIB KHALID, MD • *Washington University School of Medicine, St. Louis, MO*

JACQUELINE M. LAURIN, MD • *Georgetown University School of Medicine, Washington, DC*

KONSTANTINOS N. LAZARIDIS, MD • *Mayo Clinic, Rochester, MN*

CYNTHIA LEVY, MD • *University of Florida, Gainesville, FL*

KEITH D. LINDOR, MD • *Mayo Clinic, Rochester, MN*

VELIMIR A. LUKETIC, MD • *Virginia Commonwealth University Medical Center, Richmond, VA*

TIMOTHY M. MCCASHLAND, MD • *University of Nebraska, Omaha, NE*

MARLYN J. MAYO, MD • *University of Texas Southwestern, Dallas, TX*

ABHITABH PATIL, MD • *University of Texas Southwestern, Dallas, TX*

AARON J. SMALL, MD • *Mayo Clinic, Rochester, MN*

ALASTAIR SMITH, MD • *Duke University Medical Center, Durham, NC*

JAYANT A. TALWALKAR, MD • *Mayo Clinic, Rochester, MN*

KYMBERLY D. S. WATT, MD • *Mayo Clinic, Rochester, MN*

1 Diagnosis of Cholestasis

Velimir A. Luketic

CONTENTS

Abstract

An elevated serum alkaline phosphatase level is the hallmark of cholestasis. An abnormal gamma glutamyl transferase, 5'-nucleotidase, or liver alkaline phosphatase isoenzyme can confirm the source to be liver. Ultrasound is the most convenient way to differentiate between intrahepatic and extrahepatic cholestasis. Computed tomography or magnetic resonance imaging may be the initial test depending on the clinical setting. The level of obstruction can be identified by cholangiography: magnetic resonance cholangiography (or computed tomography cholangiogram if there are contraindications) for diagnosis alone; endoscopic retrograde cholangiography (or percutaneous transhepatic cholangiogram) if an intervention is anticipated. Endoscopic ultrasound and intraductal ultrasound may prove helpful in the evaluation of intraductal lesions. The choice of investigative test will depend on availability and local expertise in its use. Serologic studies and other disease markers can help make the diagnosis in an appropriate clinical setting or identify the next best diagnostic step. Liver biopsy often

From: *Clinical Gastroenterology: Cholestatic Liver Disease*
Edited by: K. D. Lindor and J. A. Talwalkar © Humana Press Inc., Totowa, NJ

remains the best way to make or confirm the diagnosis and to stage chronic cholestatic disease.

Key Words: Cholestasis; diagnosis.

1. INTRODUCTION

Cholestasis literally means "bile stoppage". The term was coined in the 1930s and initially used as an adjective, "cholestatic", to describe cirrhosis resulting from obstruction of the smallest biliary passages (if inflammation was present the term used was "cholangiolitic") *(1)*. It was an attempt to develop a general term for disorders with histologic findings of obstructive jaundice but normal extrahepatic bile ducts. It took more than 20 year for the term "cholestasis" to include any liver disorder characterized by impaired bile flow irrespective of the site — both large (extrahepatic cholestasis) and small, microscopic (intrahepatic cholestasis) duct injuries ultimately became part of the definition. This process was paralleled by the change from jaundice, a physical finding, to abnormal serum alkaline phosphatase (AP), a laboratory test, as the diagnostic hallmark for cholestasis. The association of high levels of AP and jaundice because of biliary obstruction was first demonstrated in 1933 *(2)*. Development of a reproducible laboratory method to test for AP (also in 1930s) extended these findings to show that chronic cholestatic liver disease is mostly anicteric *(1)*. Today, most patients with cholestasis are identified when an abnormal serum AP level is detected during routine blood testing or evaluation for an unrelated medical problem.

2. APPROACH TO DIAGNOSIS OF CHOLESTASIS

An approach to the diagnosis of cholestasis is outlined in Fig. 1. It begins with the identification of an abnormal serum AP and confirmation that it is of liver origin. The next step is to pinpoint the site of interference with the flow of bile. The primary objective is to show whether the ducts are or are not dilated thus differentiating between intrahepatic and extrahepatic cholestasis. This is usually accomplished radiologically with ultrasound (US), computed tomography (CT), or magnetic resonance imaging (MRI). The last step is to determine the cause of cholestasis and may include additional laboratory testing (serologies), additional imaging (cholangiography), as well as liver biopsy (with or without guidance).

The algorithm is not meant to be linear. The precise approach to an individual patient will depend on the clinical setting including patient

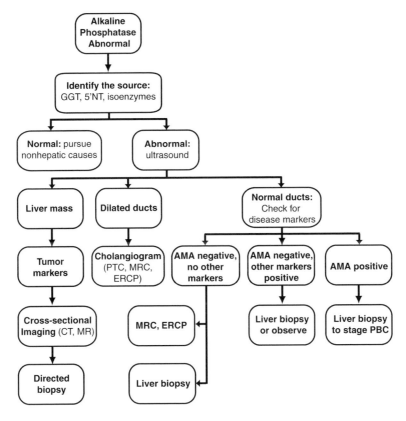

Fig. 1. Algorithm for evaluation of a cholestatic patient (see text for abbreviations).

history (family, travel, social), symptoms, and physical findings. Thus, if the patient is a middle-aged woman with pruritus and is suspected to have primary biliary cirrhosis (PBC), the initial laboratory evaluation will test not only for standard liver enzymes but also for the presence of antimitochondrial antibody (AMA) and IgM; later a liver biopsy may be indicated to stage the disease. On the other hand, the first test in a young man with ulcerative colitis will be a cholangiogram and only if it is nondiagnostic will a liver biopsy be performed. Patient history, physical examination, and laboratory testing can identify the cause in up to 90% of those with biliary obstruction *(3)*. When intrahepatic cholestasis is suspected, a thorough drug history to include over-the-counter preparations and medications taken on as-needed basis is mandatory (Table 1). Identification of an agent often requires simple observation and obviates the need for further invasive testing.

Table 1
Drugs in Current Use Reported to Cause Cholestasis (Selected List)

Anabolic steroids	Indinivir
Amoxicillin–clavulanic acid	Imipramine
Carbamazepine	Ketoconazole
Chlorpromazine	Methyltestosterone
Diltiazem	Naproxen
Erythromycin	Nevirapine
Estrogens	Phenytoin
Floxuridine	Piroxicam
Flucloxacillin	Rifampicin
Haloperidol	Total parenteral nutrition
Gold salts	Trimethoprim–sulfamethoxazole

3. CHOLESTASIS—BIOCHEMICAL ABNORMALITIES

The most sensitive test for impaired bile secretion is elevation in fasting serum bile acids *(2)*. The test is not widely available, however, and evaluation of cholestasis usually begins with detection of an elevated serum AP level. Bilirubin may or may not be elevated in cholestasis because the capacity of the liver to excrete conjugated bilirubin far exceeds the amount of pigment presented to it on a daily basis *(2)*. Aminotransferases, markers of hepatocyte injury, are rarely useful in diagnosis of cholestasis but can help with the diagnosis of an overlap syndrome.

3.1. Alkaline Phosphatase

AP catalyzes the hydrolysis of phosphate esters at an alkaline pH. Although present in nearly all tissues, clinically the most important APs are in liver, bone, kidney, and first trimester placenta. Most are coded by the same gene and differ only in posttranslation modifications characteristic of individual tissues *(4)*. Thus they are true isoenzymes. A second gene codes for intestinal and third trimester placental APs. In the liver, AP is found primarily on the surface of bile canaliculi reflecting the high AP concentrations in normal bile. In the setting of bile duct obstruction, however, the canalicular AP can be seen on the entire plasma membrane *(5)*. This reversal of polarity is thought to due to the disruption of intercellular tight junctions permitting the migration of canalicular enzymes within the hepatocyte membrane. Disruption of tight junctions between hepatocytes or cholangiocytes also permits regurgitation of bile, and thus AP, from the biliary tree via a paracellular pathway *(6)*.

Normally, serum AP reflects the activity of hepatic and bone isoenzymes. Intestinal isoenzyme can be elevated after a fatty meal in blood groups O and B *(7)*. High bone AP levels can be seen in children because of bone growth, in adults after prolonged bed rest, and in those with renal failure. In most cases, however, elevation in serum AP is a marker for liver disease, specifically, cholestasis. Increases in excess of ten times the upper limit of normal usually indicate either intra- or extrahepatic obstruction to bile flow *(8)*; lesser increases (two to three times normal) can be seen in any type of liver disorder. Clinically, a cholestatic disorder can often be differentiated from a hepatocellular disorder by the enzyme pattern: proportionally greater elevation in serum AP when compared to serum aminotransferases strongly suggests the presence of cholestasis.

3.2. Determining the Source of Alkaline Phosphatase

In as many as one-third of individuals an isolated AP elevation will not be associated with a demonstrable liver or biliary disease *(8)*. Determination of AP isoenzymes is one of the ways to identify the source of AP. Another is to measure 5′-nucleotidase, a zinc-dependent metalloenzyme present in high concentrations in the canalicular and sinusoidal membranes. Its increase parallels that of AP albeit the rise in its activity may begin after several days of cholestasis (unlike a few hours for AP) *(9)*. Since AP isoenzymes and 5′-nucleotidase are not routinely available in most clinical laboratories, a practical method to confirm liver as the source of the abnormal AP level is to test for gamma-glutamyltransferase (GGT) activity. Although present in many tissues (kidney, pancreas, spleen, lung, brain), GGT in the serum is primarily of hepatobiliary origin *(10)*. The highest GGT values are present in alcoholic liver disease, intra- and extrahepatic biliary obstruction, and in cancer infiltration of the liver. Abnormal GGT (with few exceptions, e.g., Byler's disease, benign recurrent intrahepatic cholestasis) can be seen in any hepatobiliary disorder and therefore is the least useful liver enzyme diagnostically. Since it is not found in bone, an elevated serum GGT can exclude the bone and confirm the liver as the source of elevated AP.

3.3. Aminotransferases

Aspartate (AST) and alanine (ALT) aminotransferase are intracellular enzymes that "leak" across a damaged cell membrane and abnormal serum levels are considered markers of cell injury. AST is present in both mitochondria and cytoplasm while ALT is only in the hepatocyte cytoplasm. As a result, ALT is a more specific marker of hepatocellular injury than AST. In general, ALT and AST abnormalities that are proportionately higher than ALP abnormalities are characteristic of a disease process involving hepatocytes rather than bile ducts. There are, however, exceptions. Intermittent biliary obstruction because of passage of an intraductal stone typically has AST and ALT values mimicking those seen in acute viral, toxic, or ischemic injury. During the early phases of some cholestatic disorders, e.g., intrahepatic cholestasis of pregnancy or childhood primary sclerosing cholestasis (PSC), AST and ALT are more likely to be abnormal than ALP. A mixed enzyme pattern when both AST and ALT and AP are abnormal is characteristic of an overlap syndrome with features of both autoimmune hepatitis (AIH) and a cholestatic disorder such as PBC or PSC.

3.4. Bilirubin

Bilirubin is a breakdown product of hemoglobin derived from senescent red cells. Normal serum bilirubin is largely unconjugated (indirect) (11). It is bound to serum proteins for transport to the liver where it is conjugated with glucuronide. Conjugated (direct) bilirubin is water soluble and can be secreted into bile. Hyperbilirubinemia can result from overproduction of bilirubin; decreased uptake, conjugation or excretion of bilirubin, or regurgitation of bilirubin from damaged hepatocytes or bile ducts. In extrahepatic biliary obstruction conjugated hyperbilirubinemia is present in 80% of patients (8). Whereas the proportion is less (around 50%) in those with intrahepatic cholestasis, the range is wide and the ratio of direct to indirect bilirubin is not helpful in identifying the site of obstruction. Fractionation of bilirubin is most valuable in diagnosis of disorders, mostly genetic, such as Gilbert syndrome that are characterized by unconjugated hyperbilirubinemia. The capacity of the liver to conjugate and excrete bilirubin is substantial and in most settings absolute bilirubin levels do not accurately reflect the extent of liver dysfunction. The degree of bilirubin elevation, however, is of value in determining prognosis in chronic cholestatic diseases such as PBC and PSC (12,13).

4. INTRAHEPATIC VS. EXTRAHEPATIC CHOLESTASIS—CROSS-SECTIONAL IMAGING STUDIES

Once the hepatic origin of alkaline phosphatase has been confirmed, radiologic imaging is used to identify the level of obstruction. The alternatives include intrahepatic and extrahepatic disease as well as mass

Table 2
Sensitivity and Specificity of Imaging in Obstructive Jaundice

Modality	Sensitivity (%)	Specificity (%)
US	85	80
CT	90	90
MRCP	90	97
ERCP	95	99
PTC	95	99

See text for abbreviations.
From Reddy SI and Grace ND. Liver imaging. Clin Liver Dis 2002; 6: 297–310, with permission.

effect of a space-occupying lesion. Imaging modalities include US, CT, and MRI. The choice of imaging modality will depend on the clinical situation as well as the local availability and expertise in its use.

4.1. Ultrasonography

An US examination is often the initial screening test used to evaluate cholestasis. Its advantages include wide availability, noninvasive nature, and relatively low cost. US does not expose the patient or the operator to ionizing radiation. Further, the equipment is portable and the examination can be performed at bedside without extensive preparation. There are, however, a number of limitations. US is highly dependent on the skill of the operator and the experience of the interpreter. Technical limitations include inability to penetrate bone (ribs) or air (bowel gas) interfering with the examination of the subcostal liver and subdiaphragmatic structures and the distal biliary tree and pancreas, respectively.

US is particularly good at differentiating between intrahepatic and extrahepatic biliary tract disease and identifying gallbladder pathology *(14,15)*. For optimal results the patient should be fasting in order to distend the gallbladder. In obstructive jaundice (Table 2) the sensitivity and specificity of US can exceed 80% especially if the ducts are dilated *(16)*. Because of bowel gas interference, US is less effective at determining the level of biliary obstruction or its cause (38–81%) *(16)*. For example, whereas US easily identifies gallbladder stones, a common duct stone is documented in as few as one-third of cases *(3)*. US is also quite good at detecting focal lesions within the liver *(15)*: lesions as small as 1 cm can be identified in spite of interference from extensive parenchymal disease resulting from fat or cirrhosis. US can accurately differentiate between cystic lesions (cysts, abscesses, septated cystadenomas) and solid lesions *(17)*. Because of imaging characteristics, however, it is less good at differentiating among solid hepatic masses such as hepatoma, adenoma, or focal nodular hyperplasia *(16)*. Hemangiomas have a characteristic sonographic appearance and usually require no additional evaluation. In spite of its limitations, US is an appropriate initial study in the evaluation of cholestasis because it can provide guidance and justification for further, often invasive, diagnostic testing.

4.2. Computed Tomography

Abdominal CT avoids some of the limitations of US: it is less operator dependent than US; it provides for better imaging in obese patients; and it is not prone to overlying bowel gas interference when it comes to evaluating the distal common duct and pancreas. As a consequence CT is more accurate than US at identifying the level (88–97% vs. 23–95%) as well as the cause (70–94% vs. 38–94%) of biliary obstruction if present *(16)* (Table 2). This is particularly true for pancreatic lesions and lymphadenopathy that may be responsible for extraluminal compression of the biliary tree. Paradoxically, it is less likely to identify cholesterol stones and thus is less precise at detecting choledocholithiasis *(18)*. CT scanning after bolus administration of intravenous contrast can turn an amorphous mass as seen on US into a contrast-enhanced tumor with a necrotic center. The technique can also identify vascular invasion by a tumor, an important prognostic sign. CT is better than US in identifying diffuse liver and metastatic disease and provides a more global assessment of the abdomen as a whole *(18)*. These advantages come at the expense of higher cost, radiation exposure (similar to barium enema), need for patient preparation with oral contrast, and risk of intravenous contrast allergy and renal injury. As a result, in most instances CT is reserved for evaluation of equivocal US findings, evaluation of suspected carcinoma or pancreatic abnormality, and situations where there is a need to evaluate the entire abdomen. In addition, either CT or US guidance can be used for directed biopsy of a hepatic lesion or placement of a catheter to drain an abscess.

4.3. Magnetic Resonance Imaging

Recent improvements in image acquisition techniques and use of intravenous contrast have made MRI and CT interchangeable. Advantages of MRI continue to be lack of ionizing radiation and sharp contrast resolution between normal and abnormal tissues. The disadvantages include high cost, inability to study patients with metallic devices, and blurring of images because of respiration and peristalsis.

Table 3
Causes of Extrahepatic Cholestasis

Within the lumen	Within the wall	Outside the wall
Gallstones	Primary sclerosing cholangitis	Chronic pancreatitis
Sludge	Cholangiocarcinoma	Pancreatic cancer
Microcrystals	Choledochal cyst	Lymph nodes
Parasites	Traumatic/ischemic stricture	Annular pancreas
Blood clots	Papilloma	Metastases
(hemobilia)	Carcinoid	

The latter remains a problem even with the use of newer techniques that allow for a breath-hold period of <2 s. MRI and CT are equally sensitive in the evaluation of focal nodular hyperplasia (~50% when a central scar is present), metastatic disease (36–94% for CT and 69–96% for MRI), and hepatocellular carcinoma in the setting of cirrhosis (59% for tumor mass and 37% for tumor nodule for CT and 54% for tumor mass and 55% for tumor nodule for MRI) *(19,20)*. Neither, however, can reliably distinguish between primary and metastatic tumor. In patients with cirrhosis, MRI is more sensitive than CT in distinguishing between a regenerative nodule and a tumor; neither is good at dysplastic nodules unless they are large *(21)*. MRI is the most sensitive modality for detecting cavernous hemangiomas. MRI cholangiography will be discussed later in this chapter.

5. IDENTIFYING THE CAUSE OF EXTRAHEPATIC CHOLESTASIS—CHOLANGIOGRAPHY

The use of imaging studies is designed to show whether the bile ducts are dilated thus differentiating between intrahepatic and extrahepatic cholestasis. The next step is to determine the cause and level of obstruction. Causes of extrahepatic cholestasis can be classified as those within the duct lumen, those within the duct wall, and those outside the duct. Table 3 lists some of the common causes of large duct obstruction. The gold standard for visualizing the extrahepatic biliary tree is endoscopic retrograde cholangiography (ERC). The primary advantage of ERC is that the diagnostic procedure and the therapeutic intervention can be performed at one sitting. Percutaneous transhepatic cholangiography (PTC) is reserved for patients in whom ERC is precluded for anatomic reasons or had been unsuccessful in the past. Because it is noninvasive, magnetic resonance cholangiography (MRC) is the diagnostic modality of choice when an additional therapeutic intervention is not anticipated. For those for whom MRC is contraindicated or who are unable to tolerate the procedure, CT cholagiography can be an acceptable alternative. Finally, endoscopic ultrasound (EUS) provides a low-risk way to examine the distal bile duct and surrounding structures.

5.1. Percutaneous Transhepatic Cholangiography

In PTC a percutaneous, transhepatic approach is used to inject, via a thin 22-gauge needle, contrast material into bile ducts. Sensitivity and specificity for identifying the cause and site of obstruction approaches 100% (Table 2) so long as the ducts are dilated *(22)*. When the ducts are not dilated, as in PSC, multiple attempts are often required, dramatically increasing the complication rate and decreasing the success rate to less than 80% *(23)*. Serious complications occurring in up to 3% of patients include hemobilia (4% in one series), bile peritonitis, and above all, biliary sepsis *(24)*. The latter can occur in spite of antibiotic prophylaxis especially if contrast is injected into a dilated biliary tree that had not been decompressed. In addition, if fluoroscopic rather than sonographic guidance is employed patients are exposed to ionizing radiation.

Once access to the biliary tree has been established a number of therapeutic interventions become possible. PTC has been used to document the extent of disease in PSC, balloon dilate strictures, insert an internal stent to decompress obstructed bile ducts, or obtain tissue for histologic diagnosis. Cholangiocarcinoma expands in the subepithelial layers toward the intrahepatic bile ducts and PTC is often the most effective way to obtain tissue for analysis *(25)*. Stones, sludge, as well as blood clots, can also be removed. Access to the biliary tree established by PTC can subsequently be used for endoscopic intervention ("rendezvous" technique if done at the same session). Furthermore, in patients with unresectable tumor, external drainage catheters can be left in place to decompress the biliary system.

5.2. Endoscopic Retrograde Cholangiography

In ERC endoscopic cannulation of the ampulla of Vater is used to inject contrast material to opacify the biliary tree. Once access has been obtained a number of additional diagnostic and therapeutic procedures can be performed. With the development of endoscopic sphincterotomy, ERC, initially developed as a diagnostic tool, rapidly evolved into a therapeutic one. Today the main indication for ERC is treatment rather than evaluation of suspected biliary obstruction. In part this is because the accuracy of noninvasive modalities such as MRC and EUS often rival that of ERC (Table 2). Largely, however, it is because ERC remains the most dangerous procedure routinely performed by gastroenterologists. Post-ERC pancreatitis occurs in 3–5% of purely diagnostic studies and in the largest published North American series the "any complication" (most commonly pancreatitis) rate and the procedure-related mortality after sphincterotomy were 9.8 and 0.4%, respectively *(26)*. Other procedure-associated complications include perforation, hemorrhage (after sphincterotomy), and cholangitis. In addition, patients undergoing ERC are exposed to varying amounts of ionizing radiation from fluoroscopy and spot radiography.

In skilled hands cannulation of the ampulla is almost always successful. Unlike PTC dilated bile ducts are not required for a successful ERC; a periampullary tumor, however, can prevent cannulation and precludes opacification of the biliary tree. In patients with obstructive jaundice ERC can accurately localize the level in 92–99% and identify the cause in 75–87% of cases *(27,28)*. The most common cause of extrahepatic cholestasis is choledocholithiasis *(29,30)*; after a sphincterotomy, ERC permits stone extraction via balloon or a basket and a patent sphincterotomy may prevent obstruction should another stone develop. ERC can also be used to place a nasobiliary drain to decompress an obstructed biliary tree, balloon dilate an ischemic or traumatic stricture, deploy an expandable stent across a stricture caused by a tumor, obtain brushings for cytologic evaluation from a suspected tumor, and biopsy ampullary tumors.

ERC is the standard for diagnosis of PSC. Classically, opacification of the biliary tree reveals multifocal stricturing that alternates with areas of ectasia giving the ducts a "beads-on-a-string" appearance. The changes can be intrahepatic, extrahepatic, or both (11, 2, and 87%, respectively) *(31)*. Incomplete visualization of the biliary tree because of shunting of contrast into the cystic duct and the gallbladder can be overcome by placing an inflated balloon above the cystic duct entry to perform an occlusion cholangiogram. The same technique can be used to opacify the higher-order intrahepatic ducts for a more complete examination.

One of the most difficult problems in patients with PSC is to differentiate between a dominant stricture and a cholangiocarcinoma. Since their cholangiographic appearance is quite similar, tissue confirmation is important. Techniques used include cytologic brushings, forceps biopsy, bile aspiration, or combination of all three. Recent development of thin-caliber "baby" cholangioscopes that can be introduced via the channel of a large "mother" duodenoscope permits biopsy of a suspected intraductal tumor under direct vision. Cytologic brushing of bile duct strictures is positive for cholangiocarcinoma in 30–40% of patients *(32)*. There are several reports suggesting that the combination of cytology and forceps biopsy with or without needle aspiration can increase the yield to 50–60% *(33,34)*. There is no clear evidence, however, that the improvement in yield is sufficient to justify routine use of both techniques. Thus Pugliese showed that the sensitivity of combining cytology and biopsy at 61% is only marginally better than sensitivity for either one alone at 53% *(35)*.

Diagnostic accuracy for cholangiocarcinoma may improve with expanded use of digitized image analysis (DIA) and fluorescence *in situ* hybridization (FISH), two techniques that detect cellular aneuploidy and chromosomal aberrations of suspicious tissues. DIA assesses chromatin distribution and nuclear morphology by quantifying cellular DNA. DIA was more sensitive (39.3 vs. 17.9%), and just as accurate (56 vs. 53%) albeit less specific (77.3 vs. 97.7%) than routine cytology *(36)*. FISH uses labeled DNA probes to detect chromosomal aberrations in cholangiocytes. A recent study showed FISH to be more sensitive (34 vs. 15%) and just as sensitive (97 vs. 98%) as cytology in detecting malignant strictures *(37)*.

5.3. Magnetic Resonance Cholangiography

Recent technical advances such as RARE (rapid acquisition with relaxation enhancement) and HASTE (half-Fourier-acquisition single-shot turbo spin-echo) have dramatically improved the images provided by MRC. This has been accomplished primarily by reducing the time required to take an image to a breath-hold of less than 2 s, thereby reducing motion-related artifacts. Because of the improvement in image quality and the accuracy with which bile duct abnormalities can be detected MRC has at many centers replaced ERC for diagnosis of biliary tract disease. The advantages of MRC over ERC include noninvasiveness, no ionizing radiation or iodinated contrast administration, no requirement for sedation, and less dependence on the operator. Disadvantages include patient compliance, image artifacts, lower resolution, and inability to display functional information, e.g., degree of obstruction to flow.

A recent review of 67 studies found MRC sensitivity and specificity to diagnose biliary obstruction to be 95 and 97%, respectively *(38)* (Table 2). Since the ducts are displayed in their physiologic state, MRC is a better indicator of the true ductal caliber (albeit a spasm can be mistaken for a stricture). Whereas MRC sensitivity and specificity for common bile duct stones are somewhat lower, ranging from 85 to 100% and 90 to 99%, respectively *(30)*, the overall accuracy is better than that for US or CT. As a result some have argued that patients at low risk of having a common bile duct stone should undergo MRC as the initial study,

Table 4
Sensitivity and Specificity of Magnetic Resonance Cholangiography
in Primary Sclerosing Cholangitis (PSC)

Author and reference	Patients with PSC	Sensitivity	Specificity
Fulcher, 2000 *(41)*	34*	85–88	92–97
Angulo, 2000 *(42)*	23*	83	98
Textor, 2002 *(43)*	34*†	88	99
Berstad, 2006 *(44)*	39‡	80	87

*Endoscopic retrograde cholangiopancreatography used as standard.
†Three-dimensional magnetic resonance cholangiography.
‡PSC reference standard (clinical features, biochemical profile, ERC and/or MRC, histology).
Table adapted from Stiehl A. Primary sclerosing cholangitis: the role of endoscopic therapy. Semin Liver Dis 2006; 26: 62–68, with permission, and modified with data from Berstad AE, Aabakken L, Smith H-J, Aasen S, Boberg KM, and Schrumpf E. Diagnostic accuracy of magnetic resonance and endoscopic retrograde cholangiography in primary sclerosing cholangitis. Clin Gastroenterol Hepatol 2006; 4: 514–520.

whereas those who may require a therapeutic intervention, should undergo ERC. Sensitivity is also lower for strictures, range 85–100% *(39,40)*, and for malignant conditions, 88% *(38)*. The most extensive data come from studies of patients with PSC: MRC detected PSC with a sensitivity of 80–88% and specificity of 92–99% *(41–44)* (Table 4). Since most of these studies used ERC as the standard, many authors recommend that an ERC be performed in patients at high suspicion for PSC in spite of a negative MRC. Either ERCP or MRCP can be used when both biliary and pancreatic diseases are suspected, e.g., sclerosing cholangitis in setting of autoimmune pancreatitis.

5.4. CT Cholangiography

There are a number of patients in whom MRC is contraindicated (cardiac pacemakers, metallic implants) or who cannot tolerate the procedure (claustrophobia, unable to hold breath). A reasonable noninvasive alternative in this setting is CT cholangiography. Multidetector helical CT dramatically increases the speed at which images can be obtained permitting large volumes of tissue to be scanned within a single breath-hold. Rendered images can be displayed in either two or three dimensions similar to MRI images. Early studies using either oral or intravenous cholangiographic agents suggest accuracy comparable to MRC *(30)*. The main limitations are the risk of allergic reaction and renal and/or hepatic toxicity.

5.5. Endoscopic Ultrasound

One of the limitations of conventional US (as well as CT and MRI) is adequate visualization of the distal common bile duct. The problem can be eliminated with the use of EUS since it allows placement of an US transducer in the first or second part of the duodenum. From there the biliary tree, gallbladder, adjacent vascular structures, and the peri-ampullary/pancreatic head area can be examined without interference from either bowel gas or abdominal fat. A further benefit is the ability to perform fine needle aspiration for diagnosis of biliary and pancreatic malignancy or lymphadenopathy. Sensitivity and specificity for detecting common bile duct stones are comparable to that of ERCP without the risk of pancreatitis *(30,45)*. An offshoot of EUS is intraductal US (IDUS): a small caliber US probe (~2.0 mm diameter) is passed through the channel of a standard duodenoscope directly into the bile duct. Since the probe is in a fluid medium and is close to the luminal surface, a high-frequency transducer that enhances image quality can be used. In addition to identifying ductal stones, IDUS can help distinguish between benign and malignant strictures. The sensitivity and specificity are better than EUS and especially good if ERCP tissue sampling and IDUS are combined *(46)*. Since the areas best visualized are the hilum and mid-duct, IDUS has the potential to more accurately stage cholangiocarcinoma.

6. IDENTIFYING THE CAUSE OF INTRAHEPATIC CHOLESTASIS—LABORATORY STUDIES AND LIVER BIOPSY

Some of the causes of intrahepatic cholestasis are listed in Table 5. The list is by no means exhaustive and the classification is to a certain extent arbitrary. Thus tuberculosis could also have been placed in either the system or infiltrative columns and sepsis in the infectious column heading. Prescription drugs, over-the-counter preparations, and herbal remedies are some of the most common causes of cholestasis in adults. In most patients the diagnosis can be made by taking a careful history and by excluding other causes of cholestasis. In addition to personal history, a thorough family history and a physical examination are mandatory if one hopes to diagnose familial disorders such as benign recurrent intrahepatic cholestasis, progressive familial intrahepatic cholestasis, cystic fibrosis, and sickle cell disease. The clinical setting on the other hand will help guide the workup of sepsis, benign postoperative jaundice, graft versus host disease, cholestasis resulting from

Table 5
Causes of Intrahepatic Cholestasis

Systemic	Immune mediated	Infectious	Infiltrating	Familial
Medications	Primary biliary cirrhosis	Fibrosing hepatitis	Hepatocellular carcinoma	BRIC
Hormones	Autoimmune cholangitis	Viral hepatitis	Lymphoma	PFIC (Byler's disease, etc.)
Sepsis	Graft versus host disease	AIDS cholangiopathy	Amyloid	Idiopathic adult ductopenia
Total parenteral nutrition	Allograft rejection	Tuberculosis	Metastatic malignancy	Sickle cell disease
Intrahepatic cholestasis of pregnancy	Primary sclerosing cholangitis (small duct)	Fungal infections	Sarcoidosis	Protoporphyria Cystic fibrosis

total parenteral nutrition, and intrahepatic cholestasis of pregnancy. For a number of others, however, additional laboratory testing will be required and in a significant minority the only way to make the diagnosis will be to examine the tissue obtained by liver biopsy.

6.1. Serologies

The most common chronic cholestatic liver diseases—PBC, PSC, autoimmune cholangitis (AIC)—are immune mediated and have extensive autoantibody profiles (47,48). Presence of a high AMA titer in a woman with cholestasis is virtually diagnostic of PBC; an elevated IgM immunoglobulin fraction is unique to PBC as well. Low titres of anti-nuclear (ANA) and anti-smooth muscle (ASMA) antibodies are common in PBC and PSC patients; high titres, on the other hand, and a significant elevations in AST and ALT suggest the presence of PBC/autoimmune hepatitis (AIH) overlap (47). Similarly, the same antibody and enzyme pattern in someone with PSC (often a child) raises the possibility of the PSC/AIH overlap (48). A liver biopsy with features of AIH is required for the diagnosis of PBC/AIH and PSC/AIH overlaps. Elevated ANA and ASMA in an AMA-negative patient with a cholestatic biochemical profile may indicate the presence of AIC; a biopsy showing duct destruction confirms the diagnosis.

In an acute setting, intrahepatic cholestasis may be a sign of a viral illness. Most common are infectious mononucleosis and Cytomegalovirus

(CMV), but one should never forget that hepatitis A and to a lesser extent hepatitis B can follow a primarily cholestatic, sometimes relapsing course characterized by severe pruritus. Following liver transplantation both recurrent hepatitis B and hepatitis C have presented as a rapidly progressive fibrosing cholestatic hepatitis. A high index of suspicion and appropriate testing for viral antibodies, antigens, and replication may obviate the need to perform invasive testing. Finally, all patients with cholestasis should be tested for human immunodeficiency virus (HIV) not only because of possible acquired immune deficiency syndrome (AIDS) cholangiopathy but also as a trigger to look for infiltrative disorders such as tuberculosis, *Mycobacterium avium* complex disease (MAI) and fungal infection.

6.2. Other Tests

Routine testing for markers of hemochromatosis, Wilson's disease, and α-1-antitrypsin deficiency is not indicated since these disorders rarely present as cholestasis. An abnormal angiotensin converting enzyme (ACE) level, however, could initiate a search for sarcoidosis while an elevated α-fetoprotein may direct further search for an infiltrating hepatocellular carcinoma or metastatic testicular cancer. Nonalcoholic steatohepatitis can present as an isolated elevation of AP and an abnormal glycohemoglobin may be the only indicator of its presence.

6.3. Liver Biopsy

Essentially every algorithm for evaluation of abnormal liver enzymes ultimately ends with the words "consider liver biopsy". The main reason is that liver biopsy is often the only way to make or confirm the diagnosis, identify the nature of liver injury, guide and monitor therapy, and obtain essential prognostic information. Thus after a careful laboratory, endoscopic, and radiologic evaluation, the liver biopsy may be the only way to detect an infiltrating disorder (lymphoma, sarcoidosis, metastatic carcinoma, amyloidosis), nonalcoholic fatty liver disease, small duct PSC, and idiopathic adulthood ductopenia. Similarly, confirmation of inflammatory duct injury is required for the diagnosis of acute rejection, AMA-negative PBC, or AIC. Liver biopsy is often the approach of choice in the evaluation of unexplained fever, especially in those with acquired immunodeficiency syndrome: the liver may be the only accessible organ to identify *Mycobacterium avium* complex disease, tuberculosis, histoplasmosis, and other opportunistic infections *(49)*. Biopsy confirmation is also helpful in the diagnosis of AIH overlap syndromes as well as chronic rejection after liver transplantation.

Histologic evaluation is also important in determining prognosis and as a guide to therapy. The appropriate clinical setting and an AMA or a typical cholangiogram are virtually diagnostic for PBC and PSC, respectively, and a liver biopsy is not required to make the diagnosis. Biopsy staging, however, can help identify the need for additional diagnostic measures such as US screening for hepatocellular carcinoma and endoscopic screening for varices. In addition, the extent of fibrosis can be of prognostic significance: for example, histologic staging has been used in several survival models for both PBC and PSC *(12,13)*. In drug-induced liver injury the extent of injury and the presence or absence of inflammatory infiltrate and its type can help determine prognosis (need for transplantation) and identify treatment alternatives (immunomodulators).

7. SUMMARY AND RECOMMENDATIONS

An elevated serum AP level is the hallmark of cholestasis. When other liver enzymes are also abnormal there can be little doubt that liver is the source of AP. If only AP is abnormal the quickest method to confirm liver as the source is to obtain a GGT level. US is the most convenient way to differentiate between intrahepatic and extrahepatic cholestasis. CT or MRI should be reserved for situations where the cause is thought to be a liver or pancreatic mass. Cholangiography is the preferred method to determine the level of the obstruction. If an intervention is anticipated, ERCP (or PTC) is the method of choice; for diagnosis alone MRCP should be employed unless there is a contraindication when CT cholangiogram should be performed. Newer methods still under evaluation include EUS and IDUS particularly for intraductal lesions. Local expertise and availability will often determine which modality will be used first. Serologic studies and other disease markers can help make the diagnosis in an appropriate clinical setting or identify the next best diagnostic step. Finally, liver biopsy often remains the best way to determine or confirm the diagnosis.

REFERENCES

1. McIntyre N. Cholestasis. In: Oxford Textbook of Clinical Hepatology (Bircher J, Benhamou J-P, McIntyre N, Rizetto M and Rodes J, Eds.), 2nd edn., vol 2. Oxford University Press, New York, 1999; pp. 1573–1579.
2. Rosaki SB and McIntyre N. Biochemical investigations in the management of liver disease. In: Oxford Textbook of Clinical Hepatology (Bircher J, Benhamou J-P, McIntyre N, Rizetto M and Rodes J, Eds.), 2nd edn., vol. 1. Oxford University Press, New York, 1999; pp. 503–521.

3. Burnett DA. Rational uses of hepatic imaging modalities. Semin Liver Dis 1989; 9: 1–6.
4. Posen S. Alkaline phosphatase. Ann Intern Med 1967; 67: 183–203.
5. Hagerstrand I. Distribution of alkaline phosphatase activity in healthy and diseased human liver tissue. Acta Pathol Microbiol Scand 1975; 83: 519–526.
6. Kaplan MM and Righetti A. Induction of rat liver alkaline phosphatase: the mechanism of the serum elevation in bile duct obstruction. J Clin Invest 1970; 49: 508–516.
7. Bamford KF, Harris H, Luffmana JE, et al. Serum-alkaline-phosphatase and the ABO blood groups. Lancet 1965; 1: 538–539.
8. Weisinger RA. Laboratory tests in liver disease and approach to the patient with abnormal tests. In: Textbook of Medicine (Goldman L and Bennet JC, Eds.), Saunders, Philadelphia, 2000; pp. 775–779.
9. Hill PG and Sammons HG. An assessment of 5′ nucleotidase as a liver-function test. Q J Med 1967; 36: 457–468.
10. Whitfield JB, Pounder RE, Neale G and Moss DW. Serum-glutamyl transpeptidase activity in liver disease. But 1972; 13: 702–708.
11. Billing BH. Twenty-five years of progress in bilirubin metabolism (1952–77). Gut 1978; 19: 481–491.
12. Wiesner R, Porayko MK, Dickson ER, et al. Selection and timing of liver transplantation in primary biliary cirrhosis and primary sclerosing cholangitis. Hepatology 1992; 16: 1290–1299.
13. Levy C and Lindor KD. Primary sclerosing cholangitis: epidemiology, natural history and prognosis. Semin Liver Dis 2006; 26: 22–95.
14. Pedersen OM, Nordgard K and Kvinnsland S. Value of sonography in obstructive jaundice: limitations of bile duct caliber as an index of obstruction. Scand J Gastroenterol 1987; 22: 975–981.
15. Bennett WF and Bova JG. Review of hepatic imaging and a problem-oriented approach to liver masses. Hepatology 1990; 12: 761–775.
16. Reddy SI and Grace ND. Liver imaging: a hepatologist's perspective. Clinics Liver Dis 2002; 6: 397–301.
17. Mergo PJ and Ros PR. Benign lesions of the liver. Radiol Clin North Am 1996; 36: 319–331.
18. Saini S. Imaging of the hepatobiliary tract. N Engl J Med 1997; 43: 1189–1194.
19. Kinkel K, Lu Y, Both M, et al. Detection of hepatic metastases from cancers of the gastrointestinal tract by using noninvasive methods (US, CT, MR imaging, PET): a meta-analysis. Radiology 2002; 224: 748–756.
20. Rode A, Bancel B, Douek P, et al. Small nodule detection in cirrhotic livers: evaluation with US, spiral CT and MRI and correlation with pathologic examination of explanted liver. J Comput Assist Tomogr 2001; 25: 327–336.
21. Barren RL and Peterson MS. Screening the cirrhotic liver for hepatocellular carcinoma with CT and MR imaging: opportunities and pitfalls. Radio-Graphics 2001; 21: 117–132.
22. Gold RP, Casarella WJ, Stern G, and Seaman WB. Transhepatic cholangiography: the radiologic method of choice in suspected obstructive jaundice. Radiology 1979; 133: 39–44.
23. Teplick SK, Flick P, and Brandon JC. Transhepatic cholangiography in patients with suspected biliary disease and nondilated intrahepatic bile ducts. Gastrointest Radiol 1991; 16: 193–197.
24. Savader SJ, Trerotola SO, Merine DS, et al. Hemobilia after percutaneous transhepatic biliary drainage: treatment with transcatheter embolotherapy. J Vasc Interv Radiol 1992; 3: 345–352.

25. Trambert JJ, Bron KM, Zajko JB, et al. Percutaneous transhepatic balloon dilatation of benign biliary strictures. Am J Roentgenol 1987; 149: 945–948.
26. Freeman ML, Nelson DB, Sherman S, et al. Complications of endoscopic biliary sphincterotomy. N Engl J Med 1996; 335: 909–918.
27. Peterson MS and Baron RL. Noninvasive imaging of the liver and biliary system: the role of MRI and CT in the evaluation of liver disease. In: Hepatology (Zakim D and Boyer TD, Eds.), 4th edn., vol. 1. Saunders, Philadelphia, 2003; pp. 313–341.
28. Pasanen PA, Partanen K, Pikkarainen P, et al. A comparison of ultrasound, computed tomography and endoscopic retrograde cholangiopancreatography in the differential diagnosis of benign and malignant jaundice. Eur J Surg 1993; 159: 23–29.
29. Mark DH, Flamm CR, and Aronson N. Evidence-based assessment of diagnostic modalities for common bile duct stones. Gastrointest Endosc 2002; 56(6 Suppl 2): S190–S194.
30. Baillie J, Paulson EK, and Vittellas KM. Biliary imaging: a review. Gastroenterology 2003; 124: 1686–1699.
31. Lee YM and Kaplan MM. Primary sclerosing cholangitis. N Engl J Med 1995; 332: 924–933.
32. DeBellis M, Sherman S, Fogel EL, et al. Tissue sampling at ERCP in suspected malignant biliary strictures (Part I). Gastrointest Endosc 2002; 56: 552–561.
33. Khan SA, Davidson BR, Goldin R, et al. Guidelines for the diagnosis and treatment of cholangiocarcinoma: consensus document. Gut 2002; 51(Suppl 6): VI1–VI9.
34. Franel RJ, Jin AK, Brandwein SL, et al. The combination of stricture dilatation, endoscopic needle aspiration and biliary brushings significantly improves diagnostic yield from malignant bile duct strictures. Gastrointest Endosc 2001; 54: 587–594.
35. Pugliese V, Conio M, Nicolo G, et al. Endoscopic retrograde forceps biopsy and brush cytology of biliary strictures: a prospective study. Gastrointest Endosc 1995; 42: 520–526.
36. Baron TH, Harewood GC, Rumalla A, et al. A prospective comparison of digital image analysis and routine cytology for the identification of malignancy in biliary tract strictures. Clin Gastroenterol Hepatol 2004; 2: 214–219.
37. Kipp BR, Stadheim LM, Halling SA, et al. A comparison of routine cytology and fluorescence in situ hybridization for the detection of malignant bile duct strictures. Am J Gastroenterol 2004; 99: 1675–1681.
38. Romangnuolo J, Bardou M, Rahme E, et al. Magnetic resonance cholangiopancreatography: a meta-analysis of test performance in suspected biliary disease. Ann Intern Med 2003; 139: 547–557.
39. Varghese JC, Liddell RP, Farrell MA, et al. Diagnostic accuracy of magnetic resonance cholangiopancreatography and ultrasound compared with direct cholangiography in the detection of choledocholithiasis. Clin Radiol 1999; 54: 604–614.
40. Zidi SH, Prat F, Le Guen O, et al. Performance characteristics of magnetic resonance cholangiography in the staging of malignant hilar strictures. Gut 2000; 46: 103–106.
41. Fulcher AS, Turner MA, Franklin KJ, et al. Primary sclerosing cholangitis: evaluation with MR cholangiography—a case control study. Radiology 2000; 215: 71–80.
42. Angulo P, Pearce DH, Johnson CD, et al. Magnetic resonance cholangiography in patients with biliary disease; its role in primary sclerosing cholangitis. J Hepatol 2000; 33: 520–527.

43. Textor HJ, Flacke S, Pauleit D, et al. Three-dimensional magnetic resonance cholangiopancreatography with respiratory triggering in the diagnosis of primary sclerosing cholangitis: comparison with endoscopic retrograde cholangiography. Endoscopy 2002; 34: 984–990.
44. Berstad AE, Aabakken L, Smith H-J, et al. Diagnostic accuracy of magnetic resonance and endoscopic retrograde cholangiography in primary sclerosing cholangitis. Clin Gastroenterol Hepatol 2006; 4: 514–520.
45. Kohut M, Nowakowska-Dulawa E, Marek T, et al. Accuracy of linear endoscopic ultrasonography in evaluation of patients with suspected common bile duct stones. Endoscopy 2002; 34: 299–303.
46. Farrell RJ, Agarwal B, Brandwein SL, et al. Intraductal US is a useful adjunct to ERCP for distinguishing malignant from benign biliary strictures. Gastrointest Endosc 2002; 56: 681–687.
47. Vierling JM. Primary biliary cirrhosis and autoimmune cholangiopathy. Clin Liver Dis 2004; 8: 177–194.
48. Mendes FD and Lindor KD. Primary sclerosing cholangitis. Clin Liver Dis 2004; 8: 195–211.
49. Ruijter TMG, Jan JM, Schattenker E, et al. Diagnostic value of liver biopsy in symptomatic HIV-1-infected patients. Eur J Gastroenterol Hepatol 1993; 5: 641–645.

2 Drug-Induced Cholestasis

James P. Hamilton
and Jacqueline M. Laurin

CONTENTS

Abstract

Medications and herbal supplements can induce a variety of hepatic, acute, and chronic cholestatic syndromes including bland cholestasis, cholestasis with concurrent hepatitis, bile duct injury, and extrahepatic biliary strictures and stones. Most cases of drug- and herbal-induced cholestasis are benign, but progression to chronic liver disease, cirrhosis, and death is well described. We discuss the different types of cholestasis that can be induced by medications and herbal supplements and the mechanisms of cholestasis caused by medications. We also provide some insights into treatment. In addition, specific examples of medications and herbal supplements that are known to cause one of the cholestatic syndromes are provided.

Key Words: Drug-induced cholestasis; medication-induced cholestasis; herbal-induced cholestasis; cholestatic hepatitis; vanishing bile duct syndrome.

From: *Clinical Gastroenterology: Cholestatic Liver Disease*
Edited by: K. D. Lindor and J. A. Talwalkar © Humana Press Inc., Totowa, NJ

1. BACKGROUND

Cholestasis, defined as the abnormal secretion of bile from the liver to the duodenum, may often be the result of medications or herbal supplements. The spectrum of medication-induced cholestasis may range from an acute reversible cholestasis to a chronic irreversible destruction of the bile ducts. The diagnosis of this iatrogenic condition requires the acquisition of a detailed history and a high clinical suspicion. The true incidence and prevalence of medication-induced cholestasis is unknown. Medications are implicated in 2–5% of cases of jaundice requiring hospital admission *(1)*. In a Danish study of 1100 cases of drug-induced liver disease, 178 (16%) presented with cholestasis *(2)*. Medications from virtually all pharmacologic classes and many herbal products can cause cholestasis (*see* Table 1).

Cholestasis caused by medications should be first divided into acute and chronic forms. Acute cholestasis caused by medications can present as three different clinical entities that are based on histologic findings. *Bland cholestasis* is the result of abnormal biliary secretion and is not accompanied by hepatocellular damage. *Cholestatic hepatitis* refers to cholestasis with concomitant hepatic parenchymal damage. The third form of acute cholestasis is defined by the presence of bile duct injury or *cholangiolitis*. Medications may cause chronic cholestasis through two additional mechanisms: through the obliteration of bile ducts, also known as the *vanishing bile duct syndrome*, or by extrahepatic biliary obstruction, such as *sclerosing cholangitis* and medication-induced cholelithiasis *(3,4)*. It should also be recognized that a particular medication may cause cholestasis by more than one of the preceding mechanisms.

Because the liver is responsible for concentrating and metabolizing a majority of medications, it is a prime target for medication-induced damage. The hepatic drug-metabolizing processes are hydroxylation, oxidation, reduction, or conjugation. Genetic variation in the activity of the enzymes responsible for these metabolic processes may result in a predisposition of certain individuals to develop drug-induced cholestasis. Other factors, such as age and gender, may also be important predisposing factors. Furthermore, many medications may interfere with the transport of bilirubin. Although this functional impairment of transport may result in hyperbilirubinemia, it does not cause cholestasis.

Table 1
Selected Medications and Herbal Products that Cause Cholestasis

Bland cholestasis	Cholestatic hepatitis	Cholangiolitis	Vanishing bile duct syndrome
Anabolic steroids *(32)*	Amoxicillin–clavulonic acid *(47)*	Ajmaline *(13)*	Aceprometazine *(13)*
Azathioprine *(25)*	Azathioprine	Arsenic *(13)*	Ajmaline *(13)*
Celecoxib *(88)*	Azythromycin *(92)*	Allopurinol *(13)*	Amineptine *(13)*
Cyclosporine A *(13)*	Benzodiazepines *(13)*	Amoxicillin–clavulonic acid *(45)*	Amoxicillin–clavulonic acid *(45)*
Fosinopril *(13)*	Carbamazapine *(93)*	Ampicillin *(13)*	Ampicillin *(13)*
Heparin *(25)*	Cascara *(71)*	Azathioprine *(13)*	Azathioprine *(25)*
Infliximab *(89)*	Chaparral *(73)*	Barbiturates *(13)*	Barbiturates *(13)*
Oral contraceptives *(90)*	Chlorpromazine *(25)*	Carbamazapine *(25)*	Carbamazapine *(93)*
Senna *(91)*	Chlorpropamide *(25)*	Chlorpromazine *(25)*	Carbutamide *(13)*
Tamoxifen *(13)*	Clarithromycin *(94)*	Chlorpropamide *(25)*	Chlorothiazide *(13)*
Warfarin *(25)*	Comfrey *(76)*	Clindamycin *(33)*	Chlorpromazine *(60)*
	Cyclosporine A *(13)*	Flucloxacillin *(25)*	Cimetidine *(25)*
	Danazol *(32)*	Phenytoin *(13)*	Ciprofloxacin *(52)*
	Dapsone *(13)*	Trimethoprine–sulfamethoxazole *(33)*	Clindamycin *(33)*
	Dicloxacillin *(47)*	Terfenadine *(13)*	Co-trimoxazole *(13)*
	Erythromycin *(49)*		Cyamemazine *(13)*
	Flucloxacillin *(13)*		Cyclohexyl-propionate *(13)*
	Glimepiride *(65)*		Cyproheptadine *(13)*
	Glyburide *(25)*		Erythromycin *(13)*
	Griseofulvin *(95)*		Flucloxacillin *(13)*
	Gold *(25)*		Glibenclamide *(13)*
	Greater Celandine *(77)*		Glycyrrhizin *(13)*
	Itraconazole *(96)*		Haloperidol *(13)*

(*Continued*)

Table 1 *(Continued)*

Bland cholestasis	Cholestatic hepatitis	Cholangiolitis	Vanishing bile duct syndrome
	Ketoconazole *(97)*		Ibuprofen *(19)*
	Kava *(79)*		Imipramine *(13)*
	Loracarbef *(13)*		Methyltesto-sterone *(32)*
	6-Mercaptopurine *(25)*		Norandro stenolone *(32)*
	Mesalamine *(25)*		Estriadol *(13)*
	Methimazole *(13)*		Phenytoin *(13)*
	Nifedipine *(13)*		Prochlorperazine *(25)*
	Nitrofurantoin *(25)*		Tenoxicam *(13)*
	Norfloxacin *(53)*		Tetracyclines *(100)*
	NSAIDs *(25)*		Thiabendazole *(101)*
	Ofloxacin *(25)*		Tiopronin *(13)*
	Oxacillin *(47)*		Tolbutamide *(25)*
	Pioglitazone *(25)*		Total parenteral nutrition *(25)*
	Propoxyphene *(25)*		Trimethoprine–sulfamethoxazole *(56)*
	Risperidone *(59)*		Troleandomycin *(13)*
	Rosiglitazone *(61)*		Xenalamine *(13)*
	Rofecoxib *(98)*		
	Roxithromycin		
	Terbinafine *(99)*		
	Tricyclic anti-depressants *(25)*		
	Trimethoprine–sulfamethoxazole *(33)*		
	Troglitazone *(61)*		

*Adapted from Ref. *(13)*.

2. NORMAL PHYSIOLOGY: HEPATIC TRANSPORT PROCESSES

A basic knowledge of hepatic transport processes is required prior to any discussion of cholestasis. As expected, drugs that interfere with these transport processes are liable to cause cholestasis.

2.1. Sinusoidal Membrane Transporters

There are transport systems at the basolateral, sinusoidal domain of the hepatocyte that facilitate the uptake of albumin-bound cations, anions, and neutral substances. These substances are eventually excreted into the bile through the canalicular membrane. Uptake is primarily regulated by ATP-dependent sodium pumps and the voltage gradients that these pumps create *(5)*. For example, the sodium-taurocholate cotransport polypeptide (NTCP) is the transporter responsible for the uptake of bile salts from hepatic sinusoids *(6)*. The organic anion transport polypeptides (OATPs), however, are sodium independent. OATPs have broad substrate specificity irrespective of the structure or electrical charge. There are at least four members of this family in the human liver (OATPA, B, C, and 8) *(5)* and these membrane-spanning transporters are responsible for the uptake of most medications from the sinusoids into the hepatocyte *(7)*. A third class of sinusoidal membrane transporter is termed the organic cation transporter (OCT1) and is responsible for the hepatic uptake of positively charged drugs and other cationic species *(5)*.

2.2. Intracellular Transport

Within the hepatocyte, there are several different mechanisms by which substrates are transported from the sinusoidal to the canalicular membranes. Compounds and molecules may be transported by binding to proteins in the cytoplasm, incorporating with the membrane of the endoplasmic reticulum, or being packaged within vesicles *(5)*. Vesicular transport is dependent on cytoplasmic microtubules and thus may be inhibited by medications that affect microtubules *(4)*.

2.3. Canalicular Membrane Transporters

On the apical surface of the hepatocyte, transport proteins are responsible for exporting a variety of compounds from the hepatocyte and thus are involved in the process of bile formation. The majority of these canalicular transporters are similar to the well-described CFTR (cystic fibrosis transmembrane conductance regulator) protein and the sulfonylurea receptor. Although much of the research and discovery of these proteins has occurred in animal knockout models, most can be extrapolated to the human liver. The major class of membrane transporters are referred to as multidrug resistance-associated proteins (MDRs, MRPs) originally named for their ability to confer drug resistance by exporting anticancer drugs out of cells *(5)*. For example, MDR1 exports amphipathic cationic drugs such as verapamil and daunorubicin *(8)*. MDR3 is responsible for exporting phospholipids into the biliary system. Homozygous deficiency of MDR3 leads to a syndrome of progressive familial cholestasis *(9)*. Patients with MDR3 mutations and intrahepatic cholestasis of pregnancy have been described *(10)*.

MRP2 is another major type of export pump on the canalicular domain of the hepatocyte. This membrane-spanning protein transports multiple organic anions including antibiotics and various drug conjugates *(5)*. Mutations in the MRP2 gene result in the Dubin–Johnson syndrome of cholestasis in humans *(11)*. Several other transporters that play a vital role in the process of bile formation have been described, such as the ATP-dependent bile salt export pump (BSEP), and the glutathione transporter.

2.4. Cholangiocytes

The cholangiocytes that line the biliary epithelium play a critical role in diluting and modifying the bile as it flows from the intrahepatic portions to the extrahepatic segments. As part of the normal physiologic response to meals, secretin is released from the duodenum into the portal circulation. Secretin then binds to the cholangiocytes which in turn activates the CFTR and results in bicarbonate secretion into the biliary canal *(12)*.

3. PATHOGENESIS OF DRUG-INDUCED CHOLESTASIS

The mechanisms by which medications precipitate cholestasis are complex and incompletely understood. Most drugs are lipophilic and enter the hepatocyte through the sinusoidal membrane. Within the hepatocyte, Phase I reactions (p450 system) and Phase II reactions (conjugation) occur in order to metabolize, detoxify, and facilitate the excretion of the medications. The toxic effects of the medications may be the result of metabolites or the drugs themselves. The pathogenesis of impaired bile flow varies between each form of drug-induced cholestasis *(13)*.

Drugs that cause pure cholestasis interfere with the sinusoidal uptake, intracellular transport, or canalicular secretion of bile. For example, in rat models, cyclosporin A and rifampicin have been shown to inhibit the function of the BSEP *(14)*. Drugs that cause cholestatic hepatitis do so through inflammation and hepatocyte injury. It has been theorized that deficiencies of transporters that are responsible for the removal of certain drugs, such as the aforementioned MDR class of proteins, may lead to toxic intracellular accumulations of drugs and drug metabolites, resulting in the destruction of the cytoskeletal elements required for bile export *(13)*. The pathogenesis of drug-induced cholangiolitis is not well described. It has been postulated that certain drugs may impair the function of the MDR3 transporter, which normally exports phospholipids into bile, thus resulting in bile salt induced damage to the cholangiocytes *(15)*. In fact, ursodeoxycholic acid (UDCA) was recently shown to increase the expression of MDR3 in humans, which may explain why this drug is beneficial in cholestatic liver diseases *(16)*. However, as of yet, there is no direct evidence that links medications with functional derangement of MDR3.

Chronic drug-induced cholestasis is often related to immune-mediated mechanisms. For example, in several case reports, the vanishing bile duct syndrome has been associated with Stevens–Johnson syndrome *(17–19)*. One theory suggests that certain drugs interact with endogenous hepatic proteins and result in an immune reaction that precipitates into an acute cholangitis *(13,20,21)*. A pathologic decrease in intracellular ATP is observed in an animal model of ischemic ductopenia, resulting in marked internalization of membrane proteins and impaired bile transport *(22)*. Cholestasis would then cause bile duct injury through bile acid mediated, Fas-dependent, cholangiocyte apoptosis *(23)*. One study demonstrated that genetic factors may predispose certain patients to develop drug-induced cholangiohepatitis. In a series of 22 patients who developed amoxicillin-clavulanic acid-induced cholestasis, the haplotype DRB1* 1501-0101-DQA1*0102-DQB1*0602 was present in 70% of affected individuals, versus in only 20% of control subjects *(24)*.

4. CLINICAL PRESENTATION AND DIAGNOSIS OF DRUG-INDUCED CHOLESTASIS

The majority of cases of drug-induced cholestasis are acute illnesses that resolve quickly after the offending medication is stopped *(25)*. The clinical symptoms are similar to other forms of cholestasis where jaundice, pruritus, and fatigue predominate. Depending on the amount of hepatocellular inflammation, anorexia, malaise, and nausea may also occur. In some circumstances, specifically with cholestasis related to erythromycin *(26)* or amoxicillin-clavulanate *(27)*, abdominal pain that is indistinguishable from acute cholecystitis may be present. There has been much speculation that immunologic mechanisms are responsible for certain forms of drug-induced cholestasis, and in support of this notion, symptoms of systemic hypersensitivity may be occasionally seen. For example, fever, rash, and eosinophilia have accompanied cases of cholestasis attributed to amoxicillin-clavulanate *(27)* and chlorpromazine *(28)*.

Certain medications may also cause chronic cholestasis, with clinical features remarkably similar to primary biliary cirrhosis (PBC). Prolonged jaundice, xanthomas, and pruritus have been described in patients taking a variety of different medications. Features that help to distinguish between PBC and drug-induced cholestasis are the lack of circulating antimitochondrial antibodies and the absence of granulomas on liver biopsy in the latter *(25)*. Whereas PBC may result in end-stage liver disease and death, chronic cholestasis caused by medications is usually reversible and considered benign.

Some forms of chronic medication-induced cholestasis are associated with destruction of the intrahepatic bile ducts. Although the clinical features of this vanishing bile duct syndrome are similar to other forms of chronic cholestasis, the ductopenia is often irreversible and may lead to cirrhosis and death *(13)*.

The diagnosis of drug-induced cholestasis requires a high clinical suspicion. Obviously, other forms of cholestasis should be eliminated. Routine testing for antimitochondrial antibodies, antismooth muscle (antiactin IgG) antibodies, antinuclear antibodies, ceruloplasmin, serum transferrin saturation, alpha-1 antitrypsin phenotype, and serologic testing for viral liver disease should be performed. In addition, extrahepatic biliary obstruction should be excluded with an ultrasound of the abdomen and/or ERCP/MRCP. The role of liver biopsy is controversial; however, it may be useful to determine potential for chronicity *(13)*. An International Consensus Conference established criteria for the diagnosis of drug-induced cholestasis. The chief recommendation was to analyze the temporal relationship between the administration of a medication and the development of symptoms and to determine the biochemical response after the potential offending agent is stopped *(29)*.

5. ACUTE CLINICAL SYNDROMES OF DRUG-INDUCED CHOLESTASIS

5.1. Bland (Canalicular) Cholestasis

Bland or pure cholestasis is a rare form of drug-induced cholestasis that does not exhibit any hepatic parenchymal damage. Patients with this drug reaction may develop nausea and malaise prior to the onset of jaundice and pruritus *(13)*. Laboratory abnormalities include dramatic hyperbilirubinemia and mild elevation in serum alkaline phosphatase. Transaminases may be minimally elevated or normal. On liver biopsy, the characteristic finding is canalicular dilation with bile casts, predominantly occurring in acinar zone 3 (centrilobular region). There is typically little or no inflammation or necrosis *(4,13)*. The classic drugs that result in cholestasis without hepatitis are the steroid hormones such as oral contraceptives *(30)*. Cases of azathioprine *(31)*, anabolic steroid *(32)*, erythromycin *(33)*, cyclosporine A *(34)*, and tamoxifen (3)-induced cholestasis have also been reported.

5.2. Cholestatic Hepatitis

This is the most common form of drug-induced cholestasis and is associated with hepatic parenchymal inflammation and hepatocyte necrosis. Patients with this disorder usually present with a prodrome of fatigue, anorexia, and nausea. Right-sided abdominal pain and jaundice typically follow. Laboratory abnormalities include elevated aminotransaminases (2–8 times the upper limit of normal), elevated alkaline phosphatase (>3 times the upper limit of normal) and hyper-bilirubinemia *(25)*. Because of this nonspecific presentation, patients with drug-induced cholestatic hepatitis may be misdiagnosed with acute cholecystitis or acute cholangitis *(13)*. This entity is often accompanied by a hypersensitivity syndrome, and eosinophils may be found on liver biopsy specimens. Other architectural features seen on biopsy are lobular disarray, lymphocytic infiltrates, and swollen hepa-tocytes with intracytoplasmic bile pigments *(4,13)*. Examples of drugs that may induce cholestatic hepatitis are amoxicillin–clavulanic acid, chlorpromazine, and isoniazid *(4,13)*.

5.3. Cholangiolitis

Cholestasis with bile duct injury describes the third form of acute drug-induced reaction called cholangiolitis or ductular cholestasis. Similar to cholestatic hepatitis, patients with cholangiolitis may present with symptoms of right upper quadrant pain, jaundice, and fever. Con-comitant Stevens–Johnson syndrome has also been described, thus patients may develop rash, peripheral eosinophilia, and renal failure *(13,35)*. Acute symptoms will generally resolve within days to weeks, but prolonged cholestasis with progression to the vanishing bile duct syndrome can occur. Laboratory abnormalities are similar to that found in cholestatic hepatitis. Classically, the liver biopsy will have bile casts, bile duct injury with neutrophilic infiltrates, scattered steatosis, and relatively normal appearing hepatocytes *(13)*. The absence of bile infarcts or bile lakes should help to distinguish this form of drug reaction from extrahepatic biliary obstruction *(25)*. Examples of commonly used drugs that can precipitate cholangiolitis are trimethoprim–sulfamethoxazole, and antiepileptics such as phenytoin, carbamazapine, and barbiturates *(13)*.

6. CHRONIC CLINICAL SYNDROMES
OF DRUG-INDUCED CHOLESTASIS

6.1. Vanishing Bile Duct Syndrome

In some rare cases, drug-induced cholestasis may progress to a chronic disease that is characterized by progressive ductopenia *(21)*. As previously stated, the clinical presentation of the vanishing bile duct syndrome is similar to PBC. Patients will complain of anorexia, fatigue, and intermittent abdominal pain. Coexisting autoimmune disorders that are common in PBC such as the Sicca syndrome are not present in drug-induced ductopenia. Physical exam findings may include xanthomas and hepatosplenomegaly *(13)*. Laboratory abnormalities are typically restricted to an elevated alkaline phosphatase, gamma-glutamyl transferase, and serum bilirubin. Aminotransaminase levels can be variable, but are usually not significantly elevated. Hyperlidemia and fat-soluble vitamin deficiencies can occur. Liver biopsy will demonstrate ductopenia, as defined by Ludwig to be a ≥50% loss of interlobular bile ducts *(36)*. Inflammation of the portal tracts and fibrosis (including cirrhosis) are also found on representative histologic sections. Numerous medications can cause the vanishing bile duct syndrome; the prototype is chlorpromazine *(13)*.

6.2. Drug-Induced Sclerosing Cholangitis

Strictures in the intra- and extrahepatic bile ducts have been described after the intra-arterial injection of chemotherapeutic agents into the liver. These strictures develop in more than half of patients treated with floxuridine, a drug that is used for hepatic metastases from carcinoid and colon cancer *(37)*. The hepatic duct and the confluence of the right and left hepatic ducts are the most common sites for stricture development. The pathologic mechanism is thought to be related to arterial ischemia, and jaundice usually occurs 3–6 mo after administration of the medication *(38)*. Clinically, patients with this type of drug reaction present in a similar fashion to those individuals with primary sclerosing cholangitis and patients can progress to cirrhosis. Scolicidal agents, such as cetrimide-chlorhexidine, that are used to sterilize hydatid cysts can also cause extrahepatic biliary ductal stricture development *(39)*.

6.3. Drug-Induced Cholelithiasis and Choledocholithiasis

Drugs that cause hemolysis can lead to pigment gallstone formation *(4)*. In addition, octreotide *(40)*, ceftriaxone *(41)*, and dipyridamole *(42)* have been reported to precipitate stone formation in the intra- and extrahepatic bile ducts. The obvious sequela of this drug reaction is increased risk for biliary obstruction and cholestasis.

7. SPECIFIC EXAMPLES
OF DRUG-INDUCED CHOLESTASIS
7.1. Oral Contraceptives

Among women who take oral contraceptive steroids, the incidence of cholestasis is approximately 1:10,000, but may be as high as 1:4000 in Scandinavia and Chile *(43)*. Patients typically present with a bland cholestatic pattern: pruritus, jaundice, and mild elevations in liver enzymes 2–3 mo after starting the drug, although a cholestatic hepatitis can occur in up to 15% of affected patients *(13)*. The estrogen component of these medications is usually the culpable agent, but cases of cholestasis because of a progesterone contraceptive have also been reported *(44)*. Detailed molecular investigation into the pathogenesis of the cholestasis of pregnancy has led to the discovery that estrogen causes cholestasis through a dose-dependent inhibition of the BSEP *(14)*. The prognosis of this drug reaction is excellent, with symptoms resolving in several days to weeks after drug withdrawal.

7.2. Penicillins

Cholestasis secondary to amoxicillin–clavulanic acid is common and can present with or without a coexisting hepatitis. One report described a patient with a 10-fold increase in serum aminotransaminases *(27)*. The risk of significant hepatic injury has been estimated at 1/100,000 patients exposed to the drug *(45)*. Symptoms of pruritus, nausea, jaundice, abdominal pain, and fatigue classically present 4–7 wk after initiating the drug *(27)*. Systemic findings such as fever, interstitial nephritis, and inflammation of the submandibular and lacrimal glands can also occur. Classic histologic findings are centrizonal cholestasis with or without bile duct injury, but granulomatous changes can be present *(45)*. Affected individuals are typically male and age over 60. Recovery after drug withdrawal can take up to 4 mo, and progression to the vanishing bile duct syndrome and even death have been reported *(25)*. The mechanism of amoxicillin–clavulanic acid induced cholestasis is thought to be related to an allergic reaction to the clavulanic acid portion of the drug *(27,46)*. Although it is uncommon, oxacillin, dicloxacillin, and flucloxacillin have been reported to cause cholestatic hepatitis *(47)*. Specifically, within the hepatocyte, flucloxacillin is broken down into several metabolites, one of which is directly toxic to the biliary epithelium *(48)*. In rare cases, the cephalosporins may induce cholestasis *(49)*, and ceftriaxone has been implicated in cases of medication-induced cholelithiasis in children *(50)*.

7.3. Macrolide Antibiotics

Erythromycin and the macrolide family are notorious for their ability to induce cholestasis and hepatic injury. In the seminal review of this topic, it was estimated that for every 2 million patients treated with erythromycin for 10 days, 5 will develop liver disease that requires hospitalization *(33)*. Men and woman are equally affected, and symptoms of nausea, abdominal pain, and jaundice usually present 5–20 d after drug exposure. This latency period may be of shorter duration in individuals with prior exposure. In certain cases, reactions to erythromycin can mimic acute cholecystitis *(13)*. Fever and rash are common and eosinophilia can occur in up to 60% of affected patients *(51)*. Periportal eosinophilic infiltrates are commonly seen on representative liver sections, as are features consistent with cholestasis. Given the presence of eosinophilia, the mechanism of erythromycin-induced cholestasis is presumed to be related to hypersensitivity, although treatment with corticosteroids does not improve symptoms or laboratory abnormalities. Clinical improvement is expected 2–5 wk after drug discontinuation, but liver enzymes may remain abnormal for up to 6 wk *(25)*. Progression to the vanishing bile duct syndrome has been described *(21)*. Cases of cholestasis have also been described in patients taking azithromycin, clarithromycin, and roxithromycin *(25)*.

7.4. Fluoroquinolones

There are reports of cholestatic hepatitis related to ciprofloxacin, norfloxacin, and otofloxacin use *(52–54)*. The clinical symptoms of rash and jaundice generally appear rapidly, within 1–2 wk of starting therapy with the drug. The incidence of the reaction is higher in HIV-positive patients. The mechanism of drug-induced injury is not clear, both hypersensitivity reactions and immune-mediated damage have been postulated *(25)*. The histology can be variable, and hepatocyte necrosis may be present. Most patients recover fully within 2–8 wk, but cases of fulminant hepatic failure and ductopenia are reported *(25)*.

7.5. Trimethoprim/Sulfamethoxazole

A variety of liver injuries including hepatitis, cholestatic hepatitis, hepatic necrosis, and fulminant hepatic failure have been described in patients taking trimethoprim/sulfamethoxazole *(55,56)*. The mechanism of action is thought to be related to a hypersensitivity reaction to the sulfa moiety. Patients with HIV are much more likely to develop a reaction to this drug *(25)*. Chronic cholestasis and progression to ductopenia requiring liver transplant has been reported *(25,57)*.

7.6. NSAIDS

Ibuprofen, sulindac, piroxicam, diclofenac, and nimesulide have all been reported to cause cholestasis. The reaction to these medications appears to be variable, with cases of bland cholestasis, cholestatic hepatitis, and acute hepatitis all reported *(25)*. Sulindac is probably the drug that results in the most cases. Fever, rash, jaundice, pruritus, and eosinophilia typically present within the first month of initiating therapy. The mechanism of damage is thought to be because of a hypersensitivity reaction. The Stevens–Johnson syndrome and progression to the vanishing bile duct syndrome was observed in a child treated with ibuprofen *(19)*. In a case series of patients treated with nimesulide, patients who developed cholestasis tended to be younger than 65 yr, male, and had features consistent with a hypersensitivity reaction on liver biopsy *(58)*. A total of 180 cases of diclofenac-associated hepatotoxicity were reported to the Federal Drug Administration, and 8% were found to have cholestatic injury. Three quarters of the patients who developed this drug reaction were women over age 65 *(59)*.

7.7. Neuroleptics

Chlorpromazine is the classic example of a drug that can induce cholestatic hepatitis. In susceptible individuals, nausea, vomiting, and anorexia develop within 1 mo of initiating therapy. Interestingly, more than 98% of affected patients will not develop jaundice. Accordingly, the serum bilirubin is usually only slightly elevated. Abnormal laboratory studies include elevated serum aminotransaminases, alkaline phosphatase, and serum total cholesterol *(13)*. Fever and eosinophilia can be seen in up to two-thirds of affected patients *(25)*. Although most patients will completely recover within 4–8 wk of drug withdrawal, a case of progressive ductopenia and cirrhosis has been reported *(60)*. Cholestatic hepatitis has also been attributed to carbamazapine, haloperidol, and risperidone. In one report, risperidone resulted in an increase in serum aminotransaminases, bilirubin, and alkaline phosphatase within days of starting therapy *(59)*. A hypersensitivity reaction was thought to be the mechanism of action. Carbamazapine has also been associated with the vanishing bile duct syndrome *(25)*.

7.8. Oral Antidiabetic Agents

The thiazolidinedione class of drugs has been associated with several instances of medication-induced cholestasis. Troglitazone was the first agent in this family of drugs and had to be removed from clinical use after multiple episodes of severe hepatotoxicity and fulminant hepatic failure. In one report, rosiglitazone was implicated as the cause of severe cholestatic hepatitis in a 56-yr-old woman *(61)*. However, this patient eventually recovered with corticosteroid treatment, a feature that is not common in drug-induced cholestasis *(25)*. Some other aspects of the case suggest that the diagnosis may have actually been related to granulomatous liver disease, and several authors have questioned that the drug was truly the offending agent in the patient's case *(25,62)*. There are a few case reports of pioglitazone-induced cholestasis. One of the patients had asymptomatic elevations of serum aminotransaminases, but two others developed biopsy-proven cholestatic hepatitis. Symptoms of cholestasis developed after 6 wk of drug therapy, and both the patient's labs and liver function returned to normal after drug discontinuation *(63,64)*. The mechanism of thiazolidinedione-induced cholestasis is not known.

The sulfonylureas have been implicated in several cases of drug-induced cholestasis. Tolbutamide, tolazamide, and glimepiride have been reported to be the cause of reversible cholestatic hepatitis *(25,65)*. One review described a case of glyburide-induced cholestatic hepatitis that progressed to liver failure and death *(66)*.

7.9. Herbal Preparations

The use of natural remedies is increasingly common in the United States *(67)*. One study estimated a 380% increase in herbal use between 1190 and 1997 *(68)*. Herbal preparations are not regulated by the Food and Drug Administration, and contrary to popular belief, the use of herbal products can result in serious adverse events *(69)*. Most herbal products are complex mixtures and may be subject to contamination by potentially dangerous substances such as heavy metals, fungal toxins, bacteria, and pesticides *(69)*. The liver is the central site for metabolism of drugs and xenobiotics and, not surprisingly, hepatotoxicity is the most frequent adverse reaction to herbal supplements *(70)*. The risk factors for herbal-induced cholestasis and hepatotoxicity are not well described because of the lack of controlled, prospective trials that conventional medications must undergo. However, from case reports, it is apparent that women are more often affected than men *(68)*. Patients may not be forthcoming about their use of herbal remedies, so the practitioner must have a high index of suspicion in order to establish a diagnosis and specifically question patients to determine if they are using herbal supplements or teas.

7.10. Rhamnus Purshiana *(Cascara Sagrada, Bitter Bark, California Buckthorn)*

Rhamnus purshiana bark is commonly used as a laxative and, unlike most herbals, is FDA approved for this purpose *(13)*. A case of severe cholestatic hepatitis complicated by portal hypertension was documented in a patient who developed right upper quadrant pain, nausea, and jaundice after only 3 d of taking the herb *(71)*. Not only did the patient have elevations in serum bilirubin, serum aminotransaminases, and alkaline phosphatase, he developed ascites and had a prolonged prothrombin time. Liver biopsy revealed severe lymphocytic, eosinophilic, and plasma cell infiltrates in the portal areas. The patients' symptoms resolved within 3 mo of herb withdrawal. The mechanism of injury is thought to be a hypersensitivity reaction *(13)*.

7.11. Lycopodium Serratum *(Jin Bu Huan)*

Jin Bu Huan has been used for centuries in China as an antispasmodic, analgesic, and sedative. Much controversy surrounded this herb when a report of three cases of acute hepatitis caused by the herb was published in 1994 *(72)*. The liver biopsy of one of the patients revealed dense periportal eosinophils, suggesting a hypersensitivity reaction. The readministration of Jin Bu Huan in two of the patients caused abrupt recurrence of symptoms. Eleven other cases of Jin Bu Huan induced hepatitis have since been reported, and four of these had a presentation consistent with cholestatic disease *(13)*. There are no published reports of progression to chronic liver disease after removal of the herb. The mechanism of injury is thought to be related to one of the components in the herbal preparation. Scientific analyses have revealed that levotetrahydropalmatine comprises about one-third of the Jin Bu Huan preparation. This compound is structurally similar to the pyrrolizidine alkaloids, which are chemicals found in certain Chinese teas that cause veno-occlusive disease of the liver *(13)*.

7.12. Larria *Species (Chaparral Leaf)*

Found in Mexico and the southwestern United States, chaparral leaf is used for a variety of ailments including the treatment of sexually transmitted diseases, inflammation, abdominal pain, and heart failure *(73)*. There are several reports of idiosyncratic cholestatic liver injury

induced by chaparral. Symptoms present within 1–3 mo after daily
ingestion and usually resolve after herb discontinuation *(13)*. There is
a report of chaparral-induced fulminant hepatitis that required liver
transplantation *(74)*. The mechanism of injury is unknown.

7.13. Teucrium Chamaedrys *(Germander)*

Germander extract can be found in herbal teas and is used as a diuretic,
antipyretic, stimulant, and treatment for gout or abdominal pain. Several
cases of germander-induced cholestasis and cholestatic hepatitis have
been reported *(75)*. Typically, patients develop nonspecific symptoms
such as anorexia, nausea, abdominal pain, and jaundice associated with
increased serum aminotransaminases. Most commonly used in France,
the hepatotoxic component of this herb is the furano-diterpinoids,
which deplete glutathione and cause hepatocyte necrosis *(67)*.

7.14. Symphytum Officinale *(Comfrey)*

The leaves of the comfrey plant can be made into a paste and used
to treat arthritis and other inflammatory conditions. In the United States,
comfrey was combined with pepsin and marketed as a digestive aid.
Subsequent analysis determined that comfrey preparations contained
pyrrolizidine alkaloids that are well known to cause hepatic veno-
occlusive disease. Several cases of severe hepatic failure have been
reported with the use of the herbal product. This led to banning of
sales of this product in Germany and Canada. Although most patients
present with either acute or chronic clinical signs of portal hypertension, hepatomegaly, and abdominal pain, some patients may present
with cholestatic features *(76)*.

7.15. Chelidonium Majus *(Greater Celandine)*

Preparations that contain greater celandine are widely used in Europe
for the treatment of irritable bowel syndrome and biliary dyskinesia.
Multiple cases of cholestatic hepatitis caused by greater celandine
have been reported *(77,78)*. Nine of these patients also had detectable
levels of serum autoantibodies, suggesting that this herbal medicine
invoked an autoimmune reaction *(68)*. However, the exact mechanism
of hepatotoxicity is not known.

7.16. Piper Methysticum *Rhizome (Kava Root)*

A ceremonial drink made from the kava root is used as a sedative
and psychotropic agent in many Polynesian cultures, including Fiji. In
industrialized nations, kava is used as an anxiolytic *(68)*. A wide range

of hepatotoxic reactions have been attributed to kava use, and among the more common is cholestatic hepatitis *(79)*.

7.17. Treatment

The cornerstone of treatment for drug-induced liver disease is removal of the offending agent. Patience is required for both the practitioner and the patient, as normalization of laboratory abnormalities and resolution of symptoms may require weeks to months.

Additional treatment of drug-induced cholestasis addresses the symptoms. Intense pruritus is common in many forms of cholestatic liver disease and can be debilitating. The pathogenesis of this pruritus remains controversial. Some authors suggest that the accumulation of bile acids in the dermis results in pruritus, whereas others have shown evidence that the production of endogenous opiates play a role *(80,81)*.

Cholestyramine, a bile acid sequestrant, is the first-line therapy for pruritus. Patients need to be instructed to avoid taking other medicines within 4 h of taking cholestyramine, as cholestyramine may bind other medications and limit their absorption *(13)*.

UDCA (ursodiol) is used in PBC and other cholestatic liver diseases to help alleviate some of the symptoms and improve laboratory parameters. There are several case reports regarding the use of UDCA in drug-induced cholestasis and clinical improvement in pruritus *(13,82, 83)*. At the molecular level, UDCA appears to costimulate the expression of the BSEP and phospholipid export pump in humans *(16)*.

Cases of refractory pruritus may be treated with hydroxyzine, diphenhydramine, rifampin, or phenobarbital. Hydroxyzine and diphenhydramine block type 1 histamine receptors. Rifampin upregulates the expression of the BSEP on the canalicular surface of the hepatocyte *(16)*. Phenobarbital has been shown to induce hepatic microsomal enzymes and facilitate drug detoxification *(84)*. In a randomized, double-blind, placebo-controlled trial, intravenous naloxone, an opioid antagonist, was given to patients with pruritus. The treatment group showed a significant reduction in scratching and had a reduction in the perception of pruritus *(85)*. In a pilot study of 16 patients, naltrexone, an oral opioid antagonist, was also effective at improving sleep, pruritus, and fatigue *(86)*. These beneficial effects of naltrexone were tempered by opiate withdrawal side effects occurring in 50% of treated patients.

Sclerosing cholangitis that results in symptomatic biliary strictures should be treated with endoscopic stent placement to insure adequate biliary drainage. In patients that progress to the vanishing bile duct syndrome and cirrhosis, liver transplantation has been successful *(13)*.

Corticosteroids have been used in cases of drug-induced cholestasis that are accompanied by a hypersensitivity syndrome. There is little evidence to suggest that these steroids are beneficial and cannot be recommended.

Patients with chronic cholestasis are at high risk for fat-soluble vitamin malabsorption, and these patients should be screened for vitamin deficiencies and receive parenteral replacement if necessary *(87)*.

8. CONCLUSIONS

Medications and herbals preparations are an important cause of cholestasis that is associated with virtually all pharmacologic classes. Most cases of drug- and herbal-induced cholestasis are benign and improve after drug withdrawal. It is important to recognize and remove the offending agent as quickly as possible to prevent the progression to chronic liver disease and/or fulminant hepatic failure. There are no definite risk factors for drug-induced cholestasis, but it has been theorized that certain individuals may be more susceptible than others based on their genetic code. Although most patients have clinical symptoms that are identical to other cholestatic diseases, some patients may present with symptoms of systemic hypersensitivity. Treatment of drug- and herbal-induced cholestasis consists of rapid drug discontinuation and supportive care targeted to alleviate unwanted symptoms.

REFERENCES

1. Ishak K. *Drug-Induced Liver Injury Pathology*. American Association for the Study of Liver Diseases Postgraduate Course: Clinical and Pathological Correlations in Liver Disease: Approaching the Next Millennium, 1998; p. 236.
2. Friis H and Andreasen PB. Drug-induced hepatic injury: an analysis of 1100 cases reported to the Danish Committee on Adverse Drug Reactions between 1978 and 1987. J Intern Med 1992; 232: 133–138.
3. Chitturi S and Farrell GC. Drug-induced cholestasis. Semin Gastrointest Dis 2001; 12: 113–124.
4. Erlinger S. Drug-induced cholestasis. J Hepatol 1997; 26 (Suppl 1): 1–4.
5. Boyer J. Bile Formation and Cholestasis. In: *Schiff's Diseases of the Liver* (Schiff ER, Sorrell MF, and Maddrey W. eds.), 9th ed., vol 1. Lippincott Williams and Wilkins, Baltimore, 2003; 135–165.
6. Hagenbuch B, Stieger B, Foguet M, Lubbert H, and Meier PJ. Functional expression cloning and characterization of the hepatocyte Na+/bile acid cotransport system. Proc Natl Acad Sci USA 2003; 88: 10,629–10,633.
7. Kullak-Ublick GA, Ismair MG, Stieger B, et al. Organic anion-transporting polypeptide B (OATP-B) and its functional comparison with three other OATPs of human liver. Gastroenterology 2001; 120: 525–533.
8. Gigliozzi A, Fraioli F, Sundaram P, et al. Molecular identification and functional characterization of Mdr1a in rat cholangiocytes. Gastroenterology 2000; 119: 1113–1122.

9. De Vree JM, Jacquemin E, Sturm E, et al. Mutations in the MDR3 gene cause progressive familial intrahepatic cholestasis. Proc Natl Acad Sci USA 1998; 95: 282–287.
10. Jacquemin E, De Vree JM, Cresteil D, et al. The wide spectrum of multidrug resistance 3 deficiency: from neonatal cholestasis to cirrhosis of adulthood. Gastroenterology 2001; 120: 1448–1458.
11. Paulusma CC, Kool M, Bosma PJ, et al. A mutation in the human canalicular multispecific organic anion transporter gene causes the Dubin-Johnson syndrome. Hepatology 1997; 25: 1539–1542.
12. Boyer JL. Bile duct epithelium: frontiers in transport physiology. Am J Physiol 1996; 270: G1–G5.
13. Levy C and Lindor KD. Drug-induced cholestasis. Clin Liver Dis 2003; 7: 311–330.
14. Stieger B, Fattinger K, Madon J, Kullak-Ublick GA, and Meier PJ. Drug- and estrogen-induced cholestasis through inhibition of the hepatocellular bile salt export pump (Bsep) of rat liver. Gastroenterology 2000; 118: 422–430.
15. Trauner M, Meier PJ, and Boyer JL. Molecular pathogenesis of cholestasis. N Engl J Med 1998; 339: 1217–1227.
16. Marschall HU, Wagner M, Zollner G, et al. Complementary stimulation of hepatobiliary transport and detoxification systems by rifampicin and ursodeoxycholic acid in humans. Gastroenterology 2005; 129: 476–485.
17. Srivastava M, Perez-Atayde A, and Jonas MM. Drug-associated acute-onset vanishing bile duct and Stevens-Johnson syndromes in a child. Gastroenterology 1998; 115: 743–746.
18. Garcia M, Mhanna MJ, Chung-Park MJ, Davis PH, and Srivastava MD. Efficacy of early immunosuppressive therapy in a child with carbamazepine-associated vanishing bile duct and Stevens-Johnson syndromes. Dig Dis Sci 2002; 47: 177–182.
19. Taghian M, Tran TA, Bresson-Hadni S, Menget A, Felix S, and Jacquemin E. Acute vanishing bile duct syndrome after ibuprofen therapy in a child. J Pediatr 2004; 145: 273–276.
20. Bissell DM, Gores GJ, Laskin DL, and Hoofnagle JH. Drug-induced liver injury: mechanisms and test systems. Hepatology 2001; 33: 1009–1013.
21. Degott C, Feldmann G, Larrey D, et al. Drug-induced prolonged cholestasis in adults: a histological semiquantitative study demonstrating progressive ductopenia. Hepatology 1992; 15: 244–251.
22. Doctor RB, Dahl RH, Salter KD, Fouassier L, Chen J, and Fitz JG. ATP depletion in rat cholangiocytes leads to marked internalization of membrane proteins. Hepatology 2000; 31: 1045–1054.
23. Jaeschke H, Gores GJ, Cederbaum AI, Hinson JA, Pessayre D, and Lemasters JJ. Mechanisms of hepatotoxicity. Toxicol Sci 2002; 65: 166–176.
24. O'Donohue J, Oien KA, Donaldson P, et al. Co-amoxiclav jaundice: clinical and histological features and HLA class II association. Gut 2000; 47: 717–720.
25. Mohi-ud-din R, and Lewis JH. Drug- and chemical-induced cholestasis. Clin Liver Dis 2004; 8: 95–132, vii.
26. Zafrani ES, Ishak KG, and Rudzki C. Cholestatic and hepatocellular injury associated with erythromycin esters: report of nine cases. Dig Dis Sci 1979; 24: 385–396.
27. Reddy KR, Brillant P, and Schiff ER. Amoxicillin-clavulanate potassium-associated cholestasis. Gastroenterology 1989; 96: 1135–1141.
28. Tapalaga D, Dumitrascu D, Coldea A, Ban A, and Dancea S. Drug induced hepatitis. Med Intern 1982; 20: 231–238.

29. Benichou C. Criteria of drug-induced liver disorders. Report of an international consensus meeting. J Hepatol 1990; 11: 272–276.
30. Lindberg MC. Hepatobiliary complications of oral contraceptives. J Gen Intern Med 1992; 7: 199–209.
31. DePinho RA, Goldberg CS, and Lefkowitch JH. Azathioprine and the liver. Evidence favoring idiosyncratic, mixed cholestatic-hepatocellular injury in humans. Gastroenterology 1984; 86: 162–165.
32. Stimac D, Milic S, Dintinjana RD, Kovac D, and Ristic S. Androgenic/Anabolic steroid-induced toxic hepatitis. J Clin Gastroenterol 2002; 35: 350–352.
33. Carson JL, Strom BL, Duff A, et al. Acute liver disease associated with erythromycins, sulfonamides, and tetracyclines. Ann Intern Med 1993; 119: 576–583.
34. Morales JM. Drug-induced hepatotoxicity. N Engl J Med 1996; 334: 864.
35. Geubel AP and Sempoux CL. Drug and toxin-induced bile duct disorders. J Gastroenterol Hepatol 2000; 15: 1232–1238.
36. Ludwig J, Wiesner RH, and LaRusso NF. Idiopathic adulthood ductopenia. A cause of chronic cholestatic liver disease and biliary cirrhosis. J Hepatol 1988; 7: 193–199.
37. Hohn D, Melnick J, Stagg R, et al. Biliary sclerosis in patients receiving hepatic arterial infusions of floxuridine. J Clin Oncol 1985; 3: 98–102.
38. Ludwig J, Kim CH, Wiesner RH, and Krom RA. Floxuridine-induced sclerosing cholangitis: an ischemic cholangiopathy. Hepatology 1989; 9: 215–218.
39. Tozar E, Topcu O, Karayalcin K, Akbay SI, and Hengirmen S. The effects of cetrimide-chlorhexidine combination on the hepato-pancreatico-biliary system. World J Surg 2005; 29: 754–758.
40. Sheehan MT and Nippoldt TB. Hepatolithiasis (intrahepatic stone) during octreotide therapy for acromegaly: a case report. Pituitary 2000; 3: 227–230.
41. Zinberg J, Chernaik R, Coman E, Rosenblatt R, and Brandt LJ. Reversible symptomatic biliary obstruction associated with ceftriaxone pseudolithiasis. Am J Gastroenterol 1991; 86: 1251–1254.
42. Sautereau D, Moesch C, Letard JC, Cessot F, Gainant A, and Pillegand B. Recurrence of biliary drug lithiasis due to dipyridamole. Endoscopy 1997; 29: 421–423.
43. Kreek MJ. Female sex steroids and cholestasis. Semin Liver Dis 1987; 7: 8–23.
44. Anand V and Gorard DA. Norethisterone-induced cholestasis. QJM 2005; 98: 232–234.
45. Larrey D, Vial T, Micaleff A, et al. Hepatitis associated with amoxycillin-clavulanic acid combination report of 15 cases. Gut 1992; 33: 368–371.
46. Garcia Rodriguez LA, Stricker BH, and Zimmerman HJ. Risk of acute liver injury associated with the combination of amoxicillin and clavulanic acid. Arch Intern Med 1996; 156: 1327–1332.
47. Hautekeete ML. Hepatotoxicity of antibiotics. Acta Gastroenterol Belg 1995; 58: 290–296.
48. Lakehal F, Dansette PM, Becquemont L, et al. Indirect cytotoxicity of flucloxacillin toward human biliary epithelium via metabolite formation in hepatocytes. Chem Res Toxicol 2001; 14: 694–701.
49. Zimmerman HJ and Lewis JH. Drug-induced cholestasis. Med Toxicol 1987; 2: 112–160.
50. Riccabona M, Kerbl R, Schwinger W, et al. Ceftriaxone-induced cholelithiasis— a harmless side-effect? Klin Padiatr 1993; 205: 421–423.
51. Lewis JH. Drug-induced liver disease. Med Clin North Am 2000; 84: 1275–1311, x.

52. Bataille L, Rahier J, and Geubel A. Delayed and prolonged cholestatic hepatitis with ductopenia after long-term ciprofloxacin therapy for Crohn's disease. J Hepatol 2002; 37: 696–699.

53. Romero-Gomez M, Suarez Garcia E, and Fernandez MC. Norfloxacin-induced acute cholestatic hepatitis in a patient with alcoholic liver cirrhosis. Am J Gastroenterol 1999; 94: 2324–2325.

54. Hautekeete ML, Kockx MM, Naegels S, Holvoet JK, Hubens H, and Kloppel G. Cholestatic hepatitis related to quinolones: a report of two cases. J Hepatol 1995; 23: 759–760.

55. Brown SJ and Desmond PV. Hepatotoxicity of antimicrobial agents. Semin Liver Dis 2002; 22: 157–167.

56. Alberti-Flor JJ, Hernandez ME, Ferrer JP, Howell S, and Jeffers L. Fulminant liver failure and pancreatitis associated with the use of sulfamethoxazole-trimethoprim. Am J Gastroenterol 1989; 84: 1577–1579.

57. Kowdley KV, Keeffe EB, and Fawaz KA. Prolonged cholestasis due to trimethoprim-sulfamethoxazole. Gastroenterology 1992; 102: 2148–2150.

58. Van Steenbergen W, Peeters P, De Bondt J, et al. Nimesulide-induced acute hepatitis: evidence from six cases. J Hepatol 1998; 29: 135–141.

59. Krebs S, Dormann H, Muth-Selbach U, Hahn EG, Brune K, and Schneider HT. Risperidone-induced cholestatic hepatitis. Eur J Gastroenterol Hepatol 2001; 13: 67–69.

60. Moradpour D, Altorfer J, Flury R, et al. Chlorpromazine-induced vanishing bile duct syndrome leading to biliary cirrhosis. Hepatology 1994; 20: 1437–1441.

61. Bonkovsky HL, Azar R, Bird S, Szabo G, and Banner B. Severe cholestatic hepatitis caused by thiazolidinediones: risks associated with substituting rosiglitazone for troglitazone. Dig Dis Sci 2002; 47: 1632–1637.

62. Novak D and Lewis JH. Drug-induced liver disease. Curr Opin Gastroenterol 2003; 19: 203–215.

63. Pinto AG, Cummings OW, and Chalasani N. Severe but reversible cholestatic liver injury after pioglitazone therapy. Ann Intern Med 2002; 137: 857.

64. May LD, Lefkowitch JH, Kram MT, and Rubin DE. Mixed hepatocellular-cholestatic liver injury after pioglitazone therapy. Ann Intern Med 2002; 136: 449–452.

65. Chounta A, Zouridakis S, Ellinas C, et al. Cholestatic liver injury after glimepiride therapy. J Hepatol 2005; 42: 944–946.

66. van Basten JP, van Hoek B, Zeijen R, and Stockbrugger R. Glyburide-induced cholestatic hepatitis and liver failure. Case-report and review of the literature. Neth J Med 1992; 40: 305–307.

67. Schuppan D, Jia JD, Brinkhaus B, and Hahn EG. Herbal products for liver diseases: a therapeutic challenge for the new millennium. Hepatology 1999; 30: 1099–1104.

68. Stickel F, Patsenker E, and Schuppan D. Herbal hepatotoxicity. J Hepatol 2005; 43: 901–910.

69. De Smet PA. Herbal remedies. N Engl J Med 2002; 347: 2046–2056.

70. Shaw D, Leon C, Kolev S, and Murray V. Traditional remedies and food supplements. A 5-year toxicological study (1991–1995). Drug Saf 1997; 17: 342–356.

71. Nadir A, Reddy D, and Van Thiel DH. Cascara sagrada-induced intrahepatic cholestasis causing portal hypertension: case report and review of herbal hepatotoxicity. Am J Gastroenterol 2000; 95: 3634–3637.

72. Woolf GM, Petrovic LM, Rojter SE, et al. Acute hepatitis associated with the Chinese herbal product jin bu huan. Ann Intern Med 1994; 121: 729–735.

73. Batchelor WB, Heathcote J, and Wanless IR. Chaparral-induced hepatic injury. Am J Gastroenterol 1995; 90: 831–833.
74. Gordon DW, Rosenthal G, Hart J, Sirota R, and Baker AL. Chaparral ingestion. The broadening spectrum of liver injury caused by herbal medications. JAMA 1995; 273: 489–490.
75. Perez Alvarez J, Saez-Royuela F, Gento Pena E, Lopez-Morante A, Velasco Oses A, and Martin-Lorente J. Acute hepatitis due to ingestion of Teucrium chamaedrys infusions. Gastroenterol Hepatol 2001; 24: 240–243.
76. Stickel F and Seitz HK. The efficacy and safety of comfrey. Public Health Nutr 2000; 3: 501–508.
77. Stickel F, Poschl G, Seitz HK, Waldherr R, Hahn EG, and Schuppan D. Acute hepatitis induced by Greater Celandine (Chelidonium majus). Scand J Gastroenterol 2003; 38: 565–568.
78. Benninger J, Schneider HT, Schuppan D, Kirchner T, and Hahn EG. Acute hepatitis induced by greater celandine (Chelidonium majus). Gastroenterology 1999; 117: 1234–1237.
79. Stickel F, Baumuller HM, Seitz K, et al. Hepatitis induced by Kava (*Piper methysticum* rhizoma). J Hepatol 2003; 39: 62–67.
80. Bergasa NV. The pruritus of cholestasis. J Hepatol 2005; 43: 1078–1088.
81. Raiford DS. Pruritus of chronic cholestasis. QJM 1995; 88: 603–607.
82. Smith LA, Ignacio JR, Winesett MP, et al. Vanishing bile duct syndrome: amoxicillin-clavulanic acid associated intra-hepatic cholestasis responsive to ursodeoxycholic acid. J Pediatr Gastroenterol Nutr 2005; 41: 469–473.
83. O'Brien CB, Shields DS, Saul SH, and Reddy KR. Drug-induced vanishing bile duct syndrome: response to ursodiol. Am J Gastroenterol 1996; 91: 1456–1457.
84. Bloomer JR and Boyer JL. Phenobarbital effects in cholestatic liver diseases. Ann Intern Med 1975; 82: 310–317.
85. Bergasa NV, Alling DW, Talbot TL, et al. Effects of naloxone infusions in patients with the pruritus of cholestasis. A double-blind, randomized, controlled trial. Ann Intern Med 1995; 123: 161–167.
86. Wolfhagen FH, Sternieri E, Hop WC, Vitale G, Bertolotti M, and Van Buuren HR. Oral naltrexone treatment for cholestatic pruritus: a double-blind, placebo-controlled study. Gastroenterology 1997; 113: 1264–1269.
87. Levy C and Lindor KD. Management of osteoporosis, fat-soluble vitamin deficiencies, and hyperlipidemia in primary biliary cirrhosis. Clin Liver Dis 2003; 7: 901–910.
88. Chamouard P, Walter P, Baumann R, and Poupon R. Prolonged cholestasis associated with short-term use of celecoxib. Gastroenterol Clin Biol 2005; 29: 1286–1288.
89. Tobon GJ, Canas C, Jaller JJ, Restrepo JC, and Anaya JM. Serious liver disease induced by infliximab. Clin Rheumatol 2006.
90. Schreiber AJ and Simon FR. Estrogen-induced cholestasis: clues to pathogenesis and treatment. Hepatology 1983; 3: 607–613.
91. Sonmez A, Yilmaz MI, Mas R, et al. Subacute cholestatic hepatitis likely related to the use of senna for chronic constipation. Acta Gastroenterol Belg 2005; 68: 385–387.
92. Chandrupatla S, Demetris AJ, and Rabinovitz M. Azithromycin-induced intra-hepatic cholestasis. Dig Dis Sci 2002; 47: 2186–2188.
93. Forbes GM, Jeffrey GP, Shilkin KB, and Reed WD. Carbamazepine hepatotoxicity: another cause of the vanishing bile duct syndrome. Gastroenterology 1992; 102: 1385–1388.

94. Fox JC, Szyjkowski RS, Sanderson SO, and Levine RA. Progressive cholestatic liver disease associated with clarithromycin treatment. J Clin Pharmacol 2002; 42: 676–680.
95. Chiprut RO, Viteri A, Jamroz C, and Dyck WP. Intrahepatic cholestasis after griseofulvin administration. Gastroenterology 1976; 70: 1141–1143.
96. Lavrijsen AP, Balmus KJ, Nugteren-Huying WM, Roldaan AC, Van't Wout JW, and Stricker BH. Hepatic injury associated with. Lancet 1992; 340: 251–252.
97. Lewis JH, Zimmerman HJ, Benson GD, and Ishak KG. Hepatic injury associated with ketoconazole therapy. Analysis of 33 cases. Gastroenterology 1984; 86: 503–513.
98. Papachristou GI, Demetris AJ, and Rabinovitz M. Acute cholestatic hepatitis associated with long-term use of rofecoxib. Dig Dis Sci 2004; 49: 459–461.
99. Burstein Z, Vildosola H, Lozano Z, Verona R, and Vargas G. Cholestatic toxic hepatitis caused by terbinafine: case report. Rev Gastroenterol Peru 2004; 24: 357–362.
100. Hunt CM and Washington K. Tetracycline-induced bile duct paucity and prolonged cholestasis. Gastroenterology 1994; 107: 1844–1847.
101. Manivel JC, Bloomer JR, and Snover DC. Progressive bile duct injury after thiabendazole administration. Gastroenterology 1987; 93: 245–249.

3 Primary Biliary Cirrhosis

Virginia C. Clark and Cynthia Levy

CONTENTS

Abstract

Primary biliary cirrhosis is a chronic progressive cholestatic liver disease that primarily targets middle-aged women. The pathogenesis is unknown, but several lines of evidence suggest genetic and environmental factors initiate an autoimmune process. Routine laboratory testing has led to the earlier detection of disease, so patients are often asymptomatic at the time of diagnosis. Initial symptoms are usually fatigue and pruritus. Signs of decompensated liver disease may eventually develop. Ursodeoxycholic acid is the only recommended treatment and may improve survival in selected patients. Prognostic models help predict natural history of the disease. Liver transplantation is the only definitive therapy once end-stage liver disease occurs.

Key Words: Primary biliary cirrhosis; natural history; pathogenesis; diagnosis; treatment; liver transplantation.

Primary biliary cirrhosis (PBC) is a chronic, progressive cholestatic liver disease. Small- and medium-sized intrahepatic bile ducts are slowly destroyed by an inflammatory process, presumably autoimmune

From: *Clinical Gastroenterology: Cholestatic Liver Disease*
Edited by: K. D. Lindor and J. A. Talwalkar © Humana Press Inc., Totowa, NJ

in nature. The end result is decreased bile secretion, fibrosis, eventually cirrhosis, and death from end-stage liver disease.

1. PATHOGENESIS

PBC is an organ-specific autoimmune disease whose pathogenesis is not well understood.

The breakdown in immune regulation likely results from complex interactions between a genetically susceptible host and an inciting, possibly environmental event or exposure that produces the autoantibody, resulting in the loss of self-tolerance. As this occurs, T and B lymphocytes are recruited to the liver and target biliary epithelial cells in the small bile ducts for destruction, ultimately leading to cholestatic liver disease.

Several lines of evidence for an underlying genetic susceptibility exist. Family studies show increased prevalence of disease in first degree relatives. In the northern UK, the relative risk of a sibling for PBC is estimated at 10.7 *(1)*. PBC also has the highest concordance rates between monozygotic twins of any autoimmune disease *(2)*.

Additional evidence includes the association between PBC and specific HLA haplotypes for MHC class II genes in certain populations *(3)*. The overall strength of association between HLA haplotype and PBC is not as strong as HLA associations found in type 1 autoimmune hepatitis and primary sclerosing cholangitis, suggesting this is only a piece of the etiologic puzzle *(4)*.

Antimitochondrial antibodies (AMAs) are present in 90–95% of patients with PBC. The primary target is pyruvate dehydrogenase complex-E2 (PDC-E2) *(5)*, which has a fairly conserved protein structure across species *(6)*. AMA from the sera of PBC patients has been shown to react with PDC-E2 from both humans and *Escherichia coli (7)*. For this reason, molecular mimicry, whereby antibodies generated during an immune response to microbial antigens crossreact with self-antigens, has been hypothesized as a source for the generation of autoantibodies in PBC. In addition to *E. coli*, other infectious agents like *Chlamydia pneumoniae (8)*, *Mycobacterium gordonae (9)*, *Helicobacter* species *(10)*, retroviral infection *(11)*, and most recently *Novosphingobium aromaticivorans (12)* have been implicated in the pathogenesis of PBC.

Because of the geographical differences in prevalence of PBC, environmental exposures are also hypothesized to contribute to the development of the disease. Xenobiotics are foreign compounds that complex with and/or structurally alter native self-proteins. The structural change may be sufficient to initiate an autoimmune response if no longer recognized as self. Long et al showed that sera from AMA-positive patients reacted against synthetic structures designed to mimic modified PDC-E2 *(13)*. Although data support multiple pathways for initiation of autoantibody formation, the specificity of the immune process for the liver cannot be as well explained. One hypothesis is that during apoptosis, biliary epithelial cells process PDC-E2 differently than other cells, thereby generating the specificity of the autoimmune reaction for the liver *(14)*.

2. EPIDEMIOLOGY

PBC is primarily a disease of middle-aged women, affecting women more often than men on average at a ratio of 10:1. The peak incidence occurs in the fifth decade of life, and it is uncommon in patients less than 25 yr *(14)*. The estimated incidence and prevalence of PBC varies based on geographical region. The best data come from population-based studies where the population is well defined, rigorous case finding methods are employed, and strict diagnostic criteria are applied. The first study from the UK reported an incidence of 5.8 per million and prevalence of 54 per million *(15)*. Subsequent studies described higher incidence rates, from 10 to 32 per million, and prevalence rates of 37 to 240 per million *(16–19)*. Investigators from Sweden report a similar incidence and prevalence to the UK *(20,21)*. The lowest reported incidences are between 2 and 3 per million and are from Estonia and Ontario, Canada *(22,23)*. In the United States, only one large population-based study has been conducted. The estimated incidence of PBC was 27 per million and prevalence was 400 per million, which are among the highest ever reported *(24)*. The incidence and prevalence of PBC has not been well established in many parts of the world, including Asia and Africa. Differences in geographical distribution and clustering of cases of PBC suggest exposure to environmental agent plays a role in the etiology of the disease *(25)*. Accordingly, a recent study from Australia showed the prevalence of PBC was significantly higher in immigrant populations than the native born *(26)*. In the first study to identify geographic factors in the United States, cases of PBC were found to cluster around Superfund toxic waste sites *(27)*, which provide more evidence for environmental factor. Smoking is also identified as a risk factor for development *(28)*, and perhaps progression of disease *(29)*, although these data require further validation.

3. CLINICAL FEATURES

3.1. Asymptomatic PBC

Patients asymptomatic at the time of diagnosis comprise anywhere from 32 to 80% of all patients (24,30–33). Typically, the diagnosis is suspected when liver chemistries obtained for other purposes show an elevated alkaline phosphatase or gamma-glutamyltranspeptidase (γGT). Other patients are identified by a positive AMA found during the evaluation of associated autoimmune diseases, such as Sjogren's syndrome, scleroderma, and thyroiditis. Asymptomatic patients have significantly lower levels of alkaline phosphatase and bilirubin as well as a less advanced histologic stage compared to symptomatic patients (33). Despite the absence of symptoms, between 11 and 20% of patients are cirrhotic when diagnosed (33–35).

3.2. Symptomatic PBC

The clinical presentation of PBC usually begins insidiously. Usually either pruritus or fatigue is the first symptom to appear. Approximately 10% of patients have right upper quadrant abdominal pain (36). Physical signs that can be present include hepatosplenomegaly, hyperpigmentation of the skin, and xanthelasma (37), all of which have been reported in asymptomatic patients as well. If the disease is advanced at the time of diagnosis, jaundice, ascites, and hepatic encephalopathy may be present.

Fatigue may be present in up to 68% of patients (38). Unlike pruritus, severity of liver disease does not correlate with fatigue, (39) but it can be debilitating when present. Among symptoms, fatigue has the strongest association with poor health-related quality of life in both US and European populations (40,41). In addition, a recent report suggests fatigue is an independent risk factor for cardiovascular death (42). The pathogenesis of fatigue is not known, but is hypothesized to have a centrally mediated mechanism. Ondansetron, a selective 5-HT3 receptor antagonist, did not reduce fatigue in PBC patients (43). Unfortunately, no effective therapy exists. Studies have been criticized because fatigue is a nonspecific symptom and difficult to study objectively. However, recently developed and validated fatigue measures should improve the ability to study this symptom (44).

Pruritus is a common early feature of PBC, affecting 60% of patients at the time of diagnosis (31). More recent studies report a lower prevalence (33–37%), likely reflecting a patient population with less advanced disease at the time of diagnosis (45,46) The pathogenesis of pruritus

Table 1
Extrahepatic Diseases Associated with PBC

Sjogren's syndrome
Scleroderma
CREST
Rheumatoid arthritis
Thyroid disease
Lupus erythematosis
Celiac sprue
Gallstones
Osteoporosis
Hyperlipidemia
Renal tubular acidosis
Pulmonary fibrosis
Ulcerative colitis

cannot be easily explained, but current theories implicate a central mechanism involving endogenous opioids *(47)*. Usually cholestyramine is initial therapy. If there is no response, rifampin and naltrexone are alternatives to consider *(48)*.

Other clinical concerns in patients with PBC include the development of hyperlipidemia and osteoporosis, which will be covered in another article in this issue. Patients are also at risk for fat-soluble vitamin deficiencies as the disease becomes more advanced, and screening is recommended when Mayo risk score is ≥5 *(49)*. Advanced age, male gender, and history of blood transfusion are independent risk factors for the development of hepatocellular carcinoma *(50)*. Screening is recommended once cirrhosis is present.

3.3. Associated Extrahepatic Diseases

Additional autoimmune diseases are highly prevalent in PBC. In a population-based PBC cohort, 53% of patients had at least one autoimmune condition. Scleroderma was the most prevalent at 8% *(51)*. Other autoimmune diseases include rheumatoid arthritis; lupus erythematosus; Sjogren's syndrome; calcinosis, Raynaud's, esophageal dysmotility, scleroderma, telangiectasias (CREST); and thyroid disease (Table 1) *(37,52)*. Celiac sprue may have an association with PBC in certain populations *(53,54)*. However, controversy regarding this association exists because of a high rate of false-positive tissue transglutaminase antibodies in PBC *(55)*. If patients present with steatorrhea, untreated celiac sprue, bacterial overgrowth from scleroderma, and pancreatic exocrine insufficiency should be ruled out before attributing symptoms to bile acid deficiency from cholestasis *(56)*. Renal tubular acidosis can be found *(57)*. Both pulmonary fibrosis and ulcerative colitis, while described, are rarely seen *(58,59)*.

4. DIAGNOSIS

The diagnosis of PBC is made from the presence of three features: detection of AMAs in the serum, elevation of liver enzymes for greater than 6 mo, with alkaline phosphatase as the predominant abnormality, and compatible histologic findings on liver biopsy.

AMAs in titers >1:40 are present in 90–97% of patients at the time of diagnosis *(24,60)*, and AMAs are a sensitive and specific test for PBC *(61)*. 'Autoimmune cholangitis' or 'AMA-negative PBC' describes patients with biochemical and histologic features consistent with PBC in the absence of AMA *(62)*. These patients have a different autoantibody profile, as they are likely to be positive for antinuclear antibodies (ANA) and/or antismooth muscle antibodies (ASMA) *(63)*. Based on a small number of patients studied, lack of AMA seropositivity does not affect outcomes of liver transplantation or treatment with ursodeoxycholic acid (UDCA) *(64)*.

Typically, alkaline phosphatase is greater than 2 times the upper limit of normal, whereas alanine aminotransferase (ALT) and aspartate aminotransferase (AST) are only minimally elevated. Bilirubin is usually normal at the time of diagnosis and only rises late in the course of disease. Elevated IgM titers and increased cholesterol levels are found in the majority of patients *(65)*. Elevated prothombin time reflects either malabsorption of vitamin K or end-stage liver disease *(56)*.

In the presence of a positive AMA and elevated alkaline phosphatase, a liver biopsy may not be necessary for diagnosis of PBC, but it can provide important information regarding stage of disease. Several histologic classification schemes separate the disease into four stages *(66,67)*, but notably, the histologic findings are patchy and nonuniform. Thus, several stages can be seen on one biopsy, and stages are assigned based on the most advanced finding. In stage 1, inflammation is contained within, but may expand, the portal triads. Lymphoplasmacytic cells predominate. The florid duct lesion, which is essentially pathognomonic for PBC, is defined by granulomatous destruction of intralobular bile ducts. Stage 2 involves ductular proliferation and extension of inflammation from the portal triads into the hepatic parenchyma. In stage 3, bridging fibrosis predominates, and ductopenia is more pronounced. Stage 4 is cirrhosis with regenerative nodules.

When evaluating a patient suspected to have PBC, extrahepatic biliary obstruction should be excluded, which can be easily accomplished with ultrasound. The differential diagnosis also includes primary sclerosing cholangitis, other granulomatous liver diseases like sarcoidosis, drug-induced cholestasis, and overlap syndromes with autoimmune hepatitis.

5. TREATMENT

5.1. Ursodeoxycholic Acid

UDCA is the only FDA approved drug for the treatment of PBC and is widely used. UDCA is a hydrophilic, dihydroxy bile acid which is normally present in human bile in low concentrations. Multiple mechanisms have been described *(68)*, and the effect may be multifactorial. Originally, the proposed hypothesis was that treatment with UDCA displaced endogenous (and more toxic) hydrophobic bile acids from the enterohepatic circulation. When given in standard doses of 13–15 mg/kg, as much as 40–50% of circulating bile acids are replaced with UDCA. With more hydrophilic bile acids around, cholangiocytes are protected from damage. Likely this is not the whole story. UDCA is postulated to have immunologic, anticholestatic, and antiapoptotic properties, which could all play a part in the mechanism of action *(69)*. UDCA is very well tolerated, but patients should be warned that modest weight gain can occur during the first 12 months of treatment *(70)*.

After initial observations in a small group of PBC patients suggested UDCA improved biochemical parameters, many placebo-controlled trials have been performed to evaluate the benefit of UDCA. Only five studies have included at least 100 patients who were on adequate doses of UDCA *(71–74)*. Despite these efforts, controversies regarding the role of UDCA in PBC still exist.

5.1.1. EFFECT OF UDCA ON LABORATORY TEST

Studies consistently demonstrate improvement in markers of inflammation (AST, ALT) and cholestasis (bilirubin, AP, γGT) while on treatment. The improvement is more pronounced in patients who start with bilirubin <2 mg/dL, and the largest portion of the decline occurs in the first 3–6 mo of treatment *(72)*. Whereas most patients have improvement in liver chemistry profiles, anywhere from 19 to 42% of those treated with UDCA have complete normalization of liver test at 2 yr *(75,76)*. When evaluating just bilirubin, response rates may be as high as 47% *(77)*. High baseline levels of AP, γGT, and bilirubin are associated with an incomplete response to UDCA. Interestingly, in the complete responders, liver histology improved significantly when compared to baseline. In the original randomized controlled trial from the Mayo group, time to treatment failure, specifically doubling of serum bilirubin, was prolonged in the UDCA group, and this held true in patients with both early and advanced disease. Since serum bilirubin is an independent marker of poor prognosis in PBC, does the improvement in bilirubin while on UDCA translate into improved clinical outcome? A survival analysis was performed on a group of patients with an elevated serum bilirubin level at baseline. When the serum bilirubin level normalized on UDCA treatment, survival was significantly longer than in patients whose bilirubin remained elevated (RR:3.5; 95%CI 1.6–7.7). Clinically, this is useful since bilirubin is easily measured and the 6-mo treatment value may predict survival *(77)*. Other investigators confirmed the prognostic importance of bilirubin while on UDCA, but also found levels started to rise at 4 yr of therapy *(75)*, suggesting response over time may be less.

5.1.2. EFFECT OF UDCA ON SYMPTOMS

Studies have not consistently shown improvement of pruritus and/ or fatigue while on UDCA treatment. Patients may have reduced risk of developing esophageal varices while on UDCA *(78)*.

5.1.3. EFFECT OF UDCA ON HISTOLOGY

Ideally, histologic improvement should be a reasonable surrogate marker of disease progression. The reported effects of UDCA on liver histology have been conflicting. In some of the UDCA groups, less piecemeal necrosis and portal inflammation were seen; in others, there was no difference *(79)*. Some differences in bile duct paucity and proliferation were also noticed. Pares et al were the first to show a significant difference in histologic stage while on UDCA. In this study, the interval between liver biopsies (mean 4.3–4.6 yr) was longer than in previous studies, and the majority of PBC cases had early stage disease. Delayed progression of histologic stage in early PBC (stages I–II) was confirmed by an analysis of paired biopsies from four clinical trials of UDCA *(80)*. Similarly, other investigators found the rate of progression to cirrhosis was less when treated with UDCA *(81)*. Statistical modeling has been used to show patients treated with UDCA had a fivefold lower progression rate from early stage disease to extensive fibrosis (7% per year vs 34% per year on placebo) *(82)*. Nevertheless, despite being treated with UDCA, some patients still progress to advanced disease *(73,83)*. Using the same statistical modeling based on paired biopsies, Corpechot et al showed the incidence of cirrhosis after 5 yr of UDCA was 4, 12, and 59%

among patients from stages I, II, and III, respectively. Independent prognostic factors for the development of cirrhosis while on therapy were bilirubin, albumin, and piecemeal necrosis *(84)*. These findings have implications on predicting who is at high risk for developing cirrhosis, and for design and analysis of future therapeutic trials. Overall, the effect UDCA has on histological changes is likely more pronounced in early stages of the disease and is the result of lack of progression of disease rather than an actual reversal of underlying damage. Whereas histologic improvement implies better clinical outcome, this correlation has yet to be directly shown.

5.1.4. EFFECT OF UDCA ON SURVIVAL

No single randomized controlled trial has demonstrated a survival benefit using UDCA versus placebo. In the five largest trials, the design was such that patients were given UDCA at doses of 13–15 mg/kg or placebo for 2 yr, with the exception of Pares et al, who had median time on treatment of 3.4 yr. Unfortunately, these studies were not sufficiently powered to detect a survival difference based on sample size, duration of therapy, and expected survival predicted by the Mayo risk score *(85)*. Several approaches have been taken to address effects on survival, including long-term observational studies, meta-analyses, and statistical modeling *(86)*. Longer-term observational data from the original trials have been published. Poupon et al showed a reduction in the risk of death or OLT (RR 0.32; 95%CI 0.14–0.74) after 4 yr of UDCA in the original treatment group *(73)*, which was confirmed by others *(86)*. The best evidence that UDCA provides a survival benefit is from a meta-analysis by Poupon et al. Using combined data from three trials, improved transplant-free survival was demonstrated after 4 yr of treatment with UDCA when compared to those only treated for 2 yr *(87)*. The study was criticized on the basis of selection bias, as not all trials using UDCA were included. Another meta-analysis with broader inclusion criteria failed to show a survival benefit with UDCA *(88)*. In turn, this meta-analysis was criticized for inclusion of studies using ineffective doses of UDCA and short-term follow-up, since these provide alternative explanations to the lack of survival benefit *(89)*. Other lines of evidence for a survival benefit from UDCA have also been reported. Observed transplant-free survival after 10 years of UDCA treatment is significantly higher than survival predicted by the Mayo risk score *(90)*. Pares et al recently reported similar results. Notably, in patients who had a biochemical response (defined as a decrease in alkaline phosphatase by >40% of baseline) to UDCA, observed survival was no different than a matched control population *(91)*. Finally, a similar outcome was predicted by Markov modeling, showing UDCA normalizes patient survival when given in early stages of the disease *(92)*. Evidence is accumulating to suggest an overall survival benefit with UDCA, but highlights the need for additional therapies for nonresponders.

5.2. Other Drugs to Modify Survival

Aside from UDCA, a variety of other agents have been studied for the treatment of PBC. Immunosuppressive drugs were the first agents investigated because of the presumed autoimmune nature of the disease. Cyclosporine showed a small benefit; however, hypertension and renal disease limited therapeutic usefulness *(93,94)*. Concern over bone loss in patients already predisposed to osteoporosis has limited study of corticosteroids *(95,96)*. Clear benefits from treatment with chlorambucil, azathioprine, or methotrexate have not been demonstrated *(97–102)* and none of these medications are recommended as monotherapy. A small study demonstrated a survival benefit with penicillamine, but this finding could not be confirmed in a larger controlled trial, and the drug was associated with major toxicities *(103,104)*. Several small trials showed biochemical improvement with colchicine, but no survival benefit was noted *(105–107)*. Because of the beneficial biochemical effects, colchicine was evaluated as part of combination therapy, which is discussed below. Pilot studies with malotilate and thalidomide have not shown biochemical improvements or clinical benefit *(108,109)*.

5.3. Combination Therapy

Drugs unsuccessful or without proven benefit as monotherapy have been studied adjunctively with UDCA. Methotrexate and colchicine do not provide additional benefit to UDCA treatment *(78,110–114)*. Short-term studies with budesonide, a glucocorticoid with limited systemic effects, show improvements in inflammation and histology when used in patients with early stages of PBC *(115,116)*. Other investigators found osteoporosis worsened and the Mayo risk score increased while on budesonide, which led to the conclusion that side effects were significant in the absence of clinical benefit *(117)*. However, these patients had more advanced disease when treated, possibly explaining their results. Budesonide deserves further investigation as a potential therapeutic agent. Silymarin, on the other hand, showed no efficacy in patients with an incomplete response to UDCA *(118)*.

5.4. New Agents and Future Therapies

New agents are needed for patients who have more advanced stages of disease where immunomodulating agents are less likely to work and for those who have an incomplete response to UDCA. Mycophenolate mofetil showed promise as a new therapy after a successful case report, but results from a pilot study were not as encouraging *(119)*. Pilot studies using fenofibrate and bezafibrate in combination with UDCA showed improvement in alkaline phosphatase and IgM levels *(120–125)*. Long-term controlled trials are needed to confirm these findings.

6. NATURAL HISTORY AND PROGNOSIS

The natural history of PBC is one of a slowly progressive process that results in liver damage, development of cirrhosis and its complications, and death without a liver transplant. In the early descriptions of the disease, most patients were symptomatic at the time of diagnosis *(126)*. Now it is more readily appreciated that the clinical spectrum of the disease is much broader. A recent large series reported only 4.5% of patients had liver failure at the time of diagnosis. In contrast, 61% of patients were asymptomatic when diagnosed with PBC *(46)*.

6.1. Asymptomatic PBC

Understanding of the natural history of asymptomatic PBC has evolved over the last several decades. Descriptions of the disease from the 1950s was mostly limited to patients who were symptomatic, jaundiced, and had significantly shortened survival from the time of diagnosis *(126)*. Subsequently, descriptions of asymptomatic PBC appeared after routine blood testing became widespread. Patients with an elevated alkaline phosphatase or a positive AMA identified during evaluation of an associated disorder had diagnostic or compatible liver histology in most cases *(127,128)*. Initially, the asymptomatic stage of PBC was not felt to impact patient survival *(20,30,34,129)*. Later, studies with longer follow-up showed better survival for asymptomatic patients than symptomatic patients, but decreased survival when compared to controls *(32,130)*.

Unlike previous studies, a large population-based study in Northern England found no difference in overall survival between asymptomatic and symptomatic patients. Interestingly, this was attributed to nonliver-related deaths in the asymptomatic group *(33)*. Upon further analysis, fewer liver-related deaths were noted in the initially asymptomatic patients.

Most patients with asymptomatic PBC will develop symptoms over time. The longest reported median follow-up period is 17.8 yr, which was in a group of patients who started with a normal alkaline phosphatase and positive AMA. Seventy-six percent developed symptoms, with 5.6 yr as the median time from a positive AMA to increased alkaline phosphatase. Of these, 17% died, but no death was liver related *(131)*. Recently, additional insight on the progression to symptoms has been reported *(46)*. Prince et al followed 770 patients with PBC for up to 28 yr (median 7.4 yr) and observed that after 20 yr, only 5% of patients remained asymptomatic. Pruritus develops in 31% of patients at 5 yr and 47% by 10 yr. Liver failure occurs in 12% at 5 yr and 24% by 10 yr, but only 7.3% of initially asymptomatic patients underwent liver transplantation *(33)*. Unfortunately, a uniform and consistent definition of asymptomatic PBC has not been used. This may explain conflicting results regarding certain prognostic factors like portal granuloma and presence of other autoimmune disease *(34,35,65)* as well as differences in survival. Additionally, features that predict who will develop symptoms have not been identified.

6.2. Symptomatic PBC

Once symptoms develop, reported survival averages between 6 and 12 yr *(32,33,52,126,129)*, with 18 yr being the longest reported survival *(130)*. The single best predictor of survival is bilirubin level. When the serum bilirubin level is consistently greater than 2 mg/dl, average survival is 4 yr. As levels increase to 6 mg/dl, survival is approximately 2 yr *(132)*. Other prognostic variables include age, hepatomegaly, ascites, albumin, prothrombin time, and advanced histologic stage *(133)*. Several mathematical models have been developed to simulate natural history of PBC and predict survival. The Mayo Clinic PBC risk score is widely used and has been validated repeatedly in independent patient populations. The calculation is based on a patient's age, serum bilirubin, prothrombin time, and presence of edema, all as independent predictor variables *(134)*. Advantages of the Mayo Risk Score are that there is no need for a liver biopsy since histology is not included as a prognostic variable, and it remains accurate when patients are on UDCA for treatment *(135,136)*. The development of esophageal varices also impacts survival, with a 65% one-year survival rate after the first bleeding episode *(137)*. Our group found that presence of varices can be accurately predicted by a platelet count of <140 and a Mayo risk score of ≥4.5, helping to better identify those patients to screen with endoscopy *(138)*.

7. LIVER TRANSPLANTATION

As PBC patients progress to end-stage liver disease, liver transplantation remains their only therapeutic option. Pruritus and fatigue usually resolve after transplantation. Osteoporosis also improves, but it may take 12 mo to see an increase in bone mass *(139)*. In addition to symptom improvement, transplantation offers patients a survival benefit when compared to expected survival rates *(140)*. In the United States, survival 5 yr post transplant is between 78 and 88% *(141,142)* and compares favorably with reported 5-yr survival rates of 78 and 79% from the UK and Canada *(143,144)*. UDCA has no impact on survival after transplantation, despite potentially delaying time to OLT so that other diseases may develop *(144,145)*. Prognostic models predict optimal timing for liver transplantation is around a Mayo risk score of 7.8 *(141)* or a bilirubin of 10 mg/dl *(146)*. Currently in the United States, timing of transplantation is dictated by the Model for End Stage Liver Disease (MELD) score, and it accurately predicts 3-mo mortality in PBC patients *(147)*.

PBC will recur in 8–32% of patients who undergo OLT, with median time to recurrence between 49 and 78 mo *(143,148–151)*. Some reports suggest tacrolimus-based immunosuppression increases risk of recurrence *(143,148,152)*, whereas others have not *(151)*. The role of UDCA in recurrent PBC is still undefined, but it may be beneficial *(150)*. However, how important histologic recurrence is to the clinical course of patients post transplant remains to be determined, since a significant impact on survival has not been shown *(153)*.

8. SUMMARY

PBC is a relatively uncommon cholestatic liver disease that affects middle-aged women. The etiology is unknown, but has many features of an autoimmune-mediated process. As inflammation destroys bile ducts and fibrosis develops, symptoms of fatigue and pruritus may occur. Eventually, cirrhosis may develop. The only approved and widely used medication is UDCA, which may improve liver biochemistries, delay progression of fibrosis, and development of esophageal varices, as well as improve survival free of liver transplantation. Additional studies are needed to find treatment options for patients who do not respond to UDCA. If complications of cirrhosis occur, liver transplantation can be pursued as definitive therapy.

REFERENCES

1. Jones D, Watt F, and Metcalf J. Familial primary biliary cirrhosis reassessed: a geographically-based population study. J Hepatol 1999; 30: 402–407.

2. Selmi C, Mayo MJ, Bach N, et al. Primary biliary cirrhosis in monozygotic and dizygotic twins: genetics, epigenetics, and environment. Gastroenterology 2004; 127(2): 485–492.

3. Gershwin ME, Ansari AA, Mackay IR, et al. Primary biliary cirrhosis: an orchestrated immune response against epithelial cells. Immunol Rev 2000; 174: 210–225.

4. Jones DEJ and Donaldson P. Genetic factors in the pathogenesis of primary biliary cirrhosis. Clin Liver Dis 2003; 7(4): 841–864.

5. Kita H, Nalbandian G, Keeffe EB, Coppel RL, and Gershwin ME. Pathogenesis of primary biliary cirrhosis. Clin Liver Dis 2003; 7(4): 821–839.

6. Yeaman S, Fussey S, and Danner D. Primary biliary cirrhosis: identification of two major M2 mitochondrial autoantigens. Lancet 1988; 1067–1070.

7. Fussey S, Guest J, and OF J. Identification and analysis of the major M2 autoantigens in primary biliary cirrhosis. Proc Natl Acad Sci USA 1988; 85(22): 8654–8658.

8. Abdulkarim AS, Petrovic LM, Kim W, Angulo P, Lloyd R, and Lindor K. Primary Biliary Cirrhosis: an infectious disease caused by Chlamydia pneumoniae? J Hepatol 2004; 40: 380–384.

9. Vilagut L, Vila J, Vinas O, et al. Cross-reactivity of anti-Mycobacterium gordonae antibodies with the major mitochondrial autoantigens in primary biliary cirrhosis. J Hepatol 1994; 21(4): 673–677.

10. Nilsson I, Lindgren S, Eriksson S, and Wadstrom T. Serum antibodies to Helicobacter hepaticus and Helicobacter pylori in patients with chronic liver disease. Gut 2000; 46(3): 410–414.

11. Xu L, Shen Z, Guo L, et al. Does a betaretrovirus infection trigger primary biliary cirrhosis? PNAS 2003; 100(14): 8454–8459.

12. Selmi C, Balkwill DL, Invernizzi P, et al. Patients with primary biliary cirrhosis react against a ubiquitous xenobiotic-metabolizing bacterium. Hepatology 2003; 38(5): 1251–1257.

13. Long SA, Quan C, Van de Wate J, et al. Immunoreactivity of organic mimeotopes of the E2 component of pyruvate dehydrogenase: connecting xenobiotics with primary biliary cirrhosis. J Immunol 2001; 167(5): 2956–2963.

14. Kaplan MM and Gershwin ME. primary biliary cirrhosis. N Engl J Med 2005; 353(12): 1261–1273.

15. Triger D. Primary biliary cirrhosis: an epidemiological study. BM J 1980; 281: 772–775.

16. Hamlyn AN, Macklon AF, and James O. Primary biliary cirrhosis: geographical clustering and symptomatic onset seasonality. Gut 1983; 24(10): 940–945.

17. Myszor M and James O. The epidemiology of primary biliary cirrhosis in northeast England: an increasingly common disease? QJM 1990; 276: 377–385.

18. Metcalf JV, Bhopal RS, Gray J, Howel D, and James OF. Incidence and prevalence of primary biliary cirrhosis in the city of Newcastle upon Tyne, England. Int J Epidemiol 1997; 26(4): 830–836.

19. James OF, Bhopal R, Howel D, Gray J, Burt AD, and Metcalf JV. Primary biliary cirrhosis once rare, now common in the united kingdom? Heptology 1999; 30(2): 390–394.

20. Eriksson S and Lindgren S. The prevalence and clinical spectrum of primary biliary cirrhosis in a defined population. Scand J Gastroenterol 1984; 19: 971–976.

21. Danielsson A, Boqvist L, and Uddenfeldt P. Epidemiology of primary biliary cirrhosis in a defined rural population in the northern part of Sweden. Heptology 1990; 11: 458–464.

22. Remmel T, Remmel H, Uibo R, and Salupere V. Primary biliary cirrhosis in Estonia. With special reference to incidence, prevalence, clinical features, and outcome. Scand J Gastroenterol 1995; 30: 367–371.

23. Witt-Sullivan H, Heathcote E, Cauch K, Blendis L, Ghent C, and Katz A. The demography of primary biliary cirrhosis in Ontario, Canada. Heptology 1990; 12: 98–105.

24. Kim WR, Lindor KD, Locke GR, III, et al. Epidemiology and natural history of primary biliary cirrhosis in a U. S. community. Gastroenterology 2000; 119(6): 1631–1636.

25. Selmi C, Invernizzi P, Zuin M, Podda M, and Gershwin ME. Genetics and geoepidemiology of primary biliary cirrhosis: following the footprints to disease etiology. Semin Liver Dis 2005; 25(3): 265–280.

26. Sood S, Gow PJ, Christie JM, and Angus PW. Epidemiology of primary biliary cirrhosis in Victoria, Australia: high prevalence in migrant populations. Gastroenterology 2004; 127(2): 470–475.

27. Ala A, Stanca CM, Bu-Ghanim M, et al. Increased prevalence of primary biliary cirrhosis near superfund toxic waste sites. Hepatology 2006; 43(3): 525–531.

28. Parikh-Patel A, Gold E, Worman H, Krivy KE, and Gershwin M. Risk factors for Primary Biliary Cirrhosis in a cohort of patients from the United States. Hepatology 2001; 33: 16–21.

29. Zein C, Beatty K, Post A, Falck-Ytter Y, and Logan L. Cigarette smoking is associated with increased severity of hepatic fibrosis in primary biliary cirrhosis. Gastroenterology 2006; 130(4 (Suppl. 2)): A-764.

30. James O, Watson AJ, and Macklon AF. Primary biliary cirrhosis - a revised clinical spectrum. Lancet 1981; 1278–1281.

31. Crowe J, Christensen E, Doniach D, Popper H, Tygstrup N, and Williams R. Early features of primary biliary cirrhosis: an analysis of 85 patients. Am J Gastroenterol 1985; 80(6): 466–468.

32. Nyberg A and Loof L. Primary biliary cirrhosis: clinical features and outcome, with special reference to asymptomatic disease. Scand J Gastroenterol 1989; 24: 57–64.

33. Prince MI, Chetwynd A, Craig WL, Metcalf JV, James OFW. Asymptomatic primary biliary cirrhosis: clinical features, prognosis, and symptom progression in a large population based cohort. Gut 2004; 53: 865–870.

34. Beswick D, Klatskin G, and Boyer JL. Asymptomatic primary biliary cirrhosis. A progress report on long-term follow up and natural history. Gastroenterology 1985; 89(2): 267–271.

35. Balasubramaniam K, Brambsch PM, Wiesner RH, Lindor KD, and Dickson ER. Diminished survival in asymptomatic primary biliary cirrhosis. Gastroenterology 1990; 98: 1567–1571.

36. Laurin JM, DeSotel CK, Jorgensen RA, Dickson ER, and Lindor KD. The natural history of abdominal pain associated with primary biliary cirrhosis. Am J Gastroenterol 1994; 89(10): 1840–1843.

37. Sherlock S and Scheuer PJ. The presentation and diagnosis of 100 patients with Primary Biliary Cirrhosis. N Engl J Med 1973; 289(13): 674–678.

38. Cauch-Dudek K, Abbey S, Stewart DE, and Heathcote EJ. Fatigue in primary biliary cirrhosis. Gut 1998; 43(5): 705–710.

39. Goldblatt J, Taylor PJ, Lipman T, et al. The true impact of fatigue in primary biliary cirrhosis: a population study. Gastroenterology 2002; 122(5): 1235–1241.

40. Poupon RE, Chrétien Y, Chazouillères O, Poupon R, and Chwalow J. Quality of life in patients with primary biliary cirrhosis. Hepatology 2004; 40(2): 489–494.

41. Stanca CM, Bach N, Krause C, et al. Evaluation of fatigue in U. S. patients with primary biliary cirrhosis. Am J Gastroenterol 2005; 100(5): 1104–1109.

42. Jones DEJ, Bhala N, Burt J, Goldblatt J, Prince M, and Newton JL. Four year follow up of fatigue in a geographically defined primary biliary cirrhosis patient cohort. Gut 2006; 55(4): 536–541.

43. Theal JJ, Toosi MN, Girlan L, et al. A randomized, controlled crossover trial of ondansetron in patients with primary biliary cirrhosis and fatigue. Hepatology 2005; 41(6): 1305–1312.

44. Jacoby A, Rannard A, Buck D, et al. Development, validation, and evaluation of the PBC-40, a disease specific health related quality of life measure for primary biliary cirrhosis. Gut 2005; 54(11): 1622–1629.

45. Talwalkar JA, Souto E, Jorgensen RA, and Lindor KD. Natural history of pruritus in primary biliary cirrhosis. Clin Gastroenterol Hepatol 2003; 1(4): 297–302.

46. Prince M, Chetwynd A, Newman W, Metcalf J, and James O. Survival and symptom progression in a geographically based cohort of patients with primary biliary cirrhosis: follow-up for up to 28 years. Gastroenterology 2002; 123: 1044–1051.

47. Bergasa NV. Pruritus and fatigue in primary biliary cirrhosis. Clin Liver Dis 2003; 7(4): 879–900.

48. Levy C and Lindor KD. Management of primary biliary cirrhosis. Curr Treat Options Gastroenterol 2003; 6(6): 493–498.

49. Levy C and Lindor KD. Management of osteoporosis, fat-soluble vitamin deficiencies, and hyperlipidemia in primary biliary cirrhosis. Clin Liver Dis 2003; 7(4): 901–910.

50. Shibuya A, Tanaka K, Miyakawa H, et al. Hepatocellular carcinoma and survival in patients with primary biliary cirrhosis. Hepatology 2002; 35(5): 1172–1178.

51. Watt FE, James OFW, and Jones DEJ. Patterns of autoimmunity in primary biliary cirrhosis patients and their families: a population-based cohort study. QJM 2004; 97(7): 397–406.

52. Christensen E, Crowe J, Doniach D, et al. Clinical pattern and course of disease in primary biliary cirrhosis based on an analysis of 236 patients. Gastroenterology 1980; 78: 236–246.

53. Sorensen HT, Thulstrup AM, Blomqvist P, Norgaard B, Fonager K, and Ekbom A. Risk of primary biliary liver cirrhosis in patients with coeliac disease: Danish and Swedish cohort data. Gut 1999; 44(5): 736–738.

54. Kingham JGC and Parker DR. The association between primary biliary cirrhosis and coeliac disease: a study of relative prevalences. Gut 1998; 42(1): 120–122.

55. Bizzaro N, Villalta D, Tonutti E, et al. IgA and IgG Tissue transglutaminase antibody prevalence and clinical significance in connective tissue diseases, inflammatory bowel disease, and primary biliary cirrhosis. Dig Dis Sci 2003; 48(12): 2360–2365.

56. Talwalkar JA and Lindor KD. Primary biliary cirrhosis. Lancet 2003; 362: 53–61.

57. Pares A, Rimola A, Bruguera M, Mas E, and Rodes J. Renal tubular acidosis in primary biliary cirrhosis. Gastroenterology 1981; 80(4): 681–686.

58. Bush A, Mitchison H, Walt R, Baron JH, Boylston AW, and Summerfield JA. Primary biliary cirrhosis and ulcerative colitis. Gastroenterology 1987; 92(6): 2009–2013.

59. Izdebska-Makosa Z and Zielinski J. Primary biliary cirrhosis in a patient with interstitial lung fibrosis. Chest 1987; 92(4): 766–767.

60. Uddenfeldt P and Danielsson A. Primary biliary cirrhosis: survival of a cohort followed for 10 years. J Intern Med 2000; 248: 292–298.
61. Leuschner U. Primary biliary cirrhosis–presentation and diagnosis. Clin Liver Dis 2003; 7(4): 741–758.
62. Heathcote EJ. Autoimmune cholangitis. Clin Liver Dis 1998; 2(2): 303–311, viii–ix.
63. Lacerda M, Ludwig J, Dickson E, Jorgensen R, and Lindor K. Antimitochondrial antibody-negative primary biliary cirrhosis. Am J Gastroenterol 1995; 90(2): 247–249.
64. Kim WR, Poterucha JJ, Jorgensen RA, et al. Does antimitochondrial antibody status affect response to treatment in patients with primary biliary cirrhosis? Outcomes of ursodeoxycholic acid therapy and liver transplantation. Hepatology 1997; 26(1): 22–26.
65. Springer J, Cauch-Dudek K, O'Rourke K, and Wanless IR. Asymptomatic primary biliary cirrhosis: a study of its natural history and prognosis. Am J Gastroenterol 1999; 94(1): 47–53.
66. Ludwig J, Dickson ER, and McDonald GS. Staging of chronic nonsuppurative destructive cholangitis (syndrome of primary biliary cirrhosis). Virchows Arch A Pathol Anat Histol 1978; 379(2): 103–112.
67. Scheuer P. Primary biliary cirrhosis. Proc R Soc Med 1967; 60(12): 1257–1260.
68. Paumgartner G and Beuers U. Ursodeoxycholic acid in cholestatic liver disease: mechanisms of action and therapeutic use revisited. Hepatology 2002; 36(3): 525–531.
69. Lazaridis KN and Lindor KD. Management of primary biliary cirrhosis: from diagnosis to end-stage disease. Curr Gastroenterol Rep 2000; 2(2): 94–98.
70. Siegel JL, Jorgensen R, Angulo P, and Lindor KD. Treatment with ursodeoxycholic acid is associated with weight gain in patients with primary biliary cirrhosis. J Clin Gastroenterol 2003; 37(2): 183–185.
71. Heathcote E, Cauch-Dudek K, Walker V, et al. The Canadian multicenter double-blind randomized controlled trial of ursodeoxycholic acid in primary biliary cirrhosis. Hepatology 1994; 19(5): 1149–1156.
72. Combes B, Carithers RJ, Maddrey W, et al. A randomized, double-blind, placebo-controlled trial of ursodeoxycholic acid in primary biliary cirrhosis. Hepatology 1995; 22(3): 759–766.
73. Poupon RE, Poupon R, Balkau B, and The U-PBCSG. Ursodiol for the long-term treatment of primary biliary cirrhosis. N Engl J Med 1994; 330(19): 1342–1347.
74. Lindor K, Dickson E, Baldus W, et al. Ursodeoxycholic acid in the treatment of primary biliary cirrhosis. Gastroenterology 1994; 106(5): 1284–1290.
75. van Hoogstraten HJ, Hansen BE, van Buuren HR, ten Kate FJ, van Berge-Henegouwen GP, and Schalm SW. Prognostic factors and long-term effects of ursodeoxycholic acid on liver biochemical parameters in patients with primary biliary cirrhosis. Dutch Multi-Centre PBC Study Group. J Hepatol 1999; 31(2): 256–262.
76. Jorgensen R, Angulo P, Dickson ER, and Lindor KD. Results of long-term ursodiol treatment for patients with primary biliary cirrhosis. Am J Gastroenterol 2002; 97(10): 2647–2650.
77. Bonnand A-M, Heathcote EJ, Lindor KD, and Poupon RE. Clinical significance of serum bilirubin levels under ursodeoxycholic acid therapy in patients with primary biliary cirrhosis. Hepatology 1999; 29(1): 39–43.

78. Lindor KD, Dickson ER, Jorgensen RA, et al. The combination of ursodeoxycholic acid and methotrexate for patients with primary biliary cirrhosis: The results of a pilot study. Hepatology 1995; 22(4): 1158–1162.
79. Chan CW, Papatheodoridis GV, Goulis J, and Burroughs AK. Ursodeoxycholic acid and histological progression in primary biliary cirrhosis. J Hepatol 2003; 39(6): 1094–1095.
80. Poupon RE, Lindor KD, Pares A, Chazouilleres O, Poupon R, and Heathcote EJ. Combined analysis of the effect of treatment with ursodeoxycholic acid on histologic progression in primary biliary cirrhosis. J Hepatol 2003; 39(1): 12–16.
81. Angulo P, Batts KP, Therneau TM, Jorgensen RA, Dickson ER, and Lindor KD. Long-term ursodeoxycholic acid delays histological progression in primary biliary cirrhosis. Hepatology 1999; 29(3): 644–647.
82. Corpechot C, Carrat F, Bonnand A-M, Poupon RE, and Poupon R. The effect of ursodeoxycholic acid therapy on liver fibrosis progression in primary biliary cirrhosis. Hepatology 2000; 32(6): 1196–1199.
83. Leuschner U, Guldutuna S, Imhof M, Hubner K, Benjaminov A, and Leuschner M. Effects of ursodeoxycholic acid after 4 to 12 years of therapy in early and late stages of primary biliary cirrhosis. J Hepatol 1994; 21(4): 624–633.
84. Corpechot C, Carrat F, Poupon R, and Poupon R-E. Primary biliary cirrhosis: Incidence and predictive factors of cirrhosis development in ursodiol-treated patients. Gastroenterology 2002; 122(3): 652–658.
85. Carithers J and Robert L. Primary biliary cirrhosis: specific treatment. Clin Liver Dis 2003; 7(4): 923–939.
86. Lindor KD, Therneau TM, Jorgensen RA, Malinchoc M, and Dickson ER. Effects of ursodeoxycholic acid on survival in patients with primary biliary cirrhosis. Gastroenterology 1996; 110(5): 1515–1518.
87. Poupon R, Lindor K, Cauch-Dudek K, Dickson E, Poupon R, and Heathcote E. Combined analysis of randomized controlled trials of ursodeoxycholic acid in primary biliary cirrhosis. Gastroenterology 1997; 113(3): 884–890.
88. Goulis J, Leandro G, and Burroughs AK. Randomised controlled trials of ursodeoxycholic-acid therapy for primary biliary cirrhosis: a meta-analysis. Lancet 1999; 354: 1053–1060.
89. Lindor KD, Poupon R, Poupon R, Heathcote EJ, and Therneau T. Ursodeoxycholic acid for primary biliary cirrhosis. Lancet 2000; 355(9204): 657–658.
90. Poupon RE, Bonnand A-M, Chrétien Y, and Poupon R. Ten-year survival in ursodeoxycholic acid-treated patients with primary biliary cirrhosis. Hepatology 1999; 29(6): 1668–1671.
91. Pares A, Caballeria L, and Rodes J. Excellent long-term survival in patients with primary biliary cirrhosis and biochemical response to ursodeoxycholic acid. Gastroenterology 2006; 130(3): 715–720.
92. Corpechot C, Carrat F, Bahr A, Chretien Y, Poupon R-E, and Poupon R. The effect of ursodeoxycholic acid therapy on the natural course of primary biliary cirrhosis. Gastroenterology 2005; 128(2): 297–303.
93. Wiesner RH, Ludwig J, Lindor KD, et al. A controlled trial of cyclosporine in the treatment of primary biliary cirrhosis. N Engl J Med 1990; 322(20): 1419–1424.
94. Lombard M, Portmann B, Neuberger J, et al. Cyclosporin A treatment in primary biliary cirrhosis: results of a long-term placebo controlled trial. Gastroenterology 1993; 104(2): 519–526.

95. Mitchison HC, Bassendine MF, Malcolm AJ, et al. A pilot, double-blind, controlled 1-year trial of prednisolone treatment in primary biliary cirrhosis: hepatic improvement but greater bone loss. Hepatology 1989; 10(4): 420–429.
96. Mitchison HC, Palmer JM, Bassendine MF, Watson AJ, Record CO, and James OF. A controlled trial of prednisolone treatment in primary biliary cirrhosis. Three-year results. J Hepatol 1992; 15(3): 336–344.
97. Hoofnagle JH, Davis GL, Schafer DF, et al. Randomized trial of chlorambucil for primary biliary cirrhosis. Gastroenterology 1986; 91(6): 1327–1334.
98. Christensen E, Neuberger J, Crowe J, et al. Beneficial effect of azathioprine and prediction of prognosis in primary biliary cirrhosis. Final results of an international trial. Gastroenterology 1985; 89(5): 1084–1091.
99. Kaplan M and Knox T. Treatment of primary biliary cirrhosis with low dose weekly methotrexate. Gastroenterology 1991; 101(5): 1332–1338.
100. Kaplan MM, DeLellis RA, and Wolfe HJ. Sustained biochemical and histologic remission of primary biliary cirrhosis in response to medical treatment. Ann Intern Med 1997; 126(9): 682–688.
101. Bergasa NV, Jones A, Kleiner DE, et al. Pilot study of low dose oral methotrexate treatment for primary biliary cirrhosis. Am J Gastroenterol 1996; 91(2): 295–299.
102. Hendrickse MT, Rigney E, Giaffer MH, et al. Low-dose methotrexate is ineffective in primary biliary cirrhosis: long-term results of a placebo-controlled trial. Gastroenterology 1999; 117(2): 400–407.
103. Epstein O. Review: the treatment of primary biliary cirrhosis. Aliment Pharmacol Ther 1988; 2(1): 1–12.
104. Dickson ER, Fleming TR, Wiesner RH, et al. Trial of penicillamine in advanced primary biliary cirrhosis. N Engl J Med 1985; 312(16): 1011–1015.
105. Kaplan MM, Alling DW, Zimmerman HJ, et al. A prospective trial of colchicine for primary biliary cirrhosis. N Engl J Med 1986; 315(23): 1448–1454.
106. Vuoristo M, Farkkila M, Karvonen AL, et al. A placebo-controlled trial of primary biliary cirrhosis treatment with colchicine and ursodeoxycholic acid. Gastroenterology 1995; 108(5): 1470–1478.
107. Kaplan MM, Schmid C, Provenzale D, Sharma A, Dickstein G, and McKusick A. A prospective trial of colchicine and methotrexate in the treatment of primary biliary cirrhosis. Gastroenterology 1999; 117(5): 1173–1180.
108. The results of a randomized double blind controlled trial evaluating malotilate in primary biliary cirrhosis. A European multicentre study group. J Hepatol 1993; 17(2): 227–235.
109. McCormick PA, Scott F, Epstein O, Burroughs AK, Scheuer PJ, and McIntyre N. Thalidomide as therapy for primary biliary cirrhosis: a double-blind placebo controlled pilot study. J Hepatol 1994; 21(4): 496–499.
110. Gonzalez-Koch A, Brahm J, Antezana C, Smok G, and Cumsille MA. The combination of ursodeoxycholic acid and methotrexate for primary biliary cirrhosis is not better than ursodeoxycholic acid alone. J Hepatol 1997; 27(1): 143–149.
111. Combes B, Emerson SS, Flye NL, et al. Methotrexate (MTX) plus ursodeoxycholic acid (UDCA) in the treatment of primary biliary cirrhosis. Hepatology 2005; 42(5): 1184–1193.
112. Poupon RE, Huet PM, Poupon R, Bonnand AM, Nhieu JT, and Zafrani ES. A randomized trial comparing colchicine and ursodeoxycholic acid combination

to ursodeoxycholic acid in primary biliary cirrhosis. UDCA-PBC Study Group. Hepatology 1996; 4(5): 1098–1103.

113. Battezzati PM, Zuin M, Crosignani A, et al. Ten-year combination treatment with colchicine and ursodeoxycholic acid for primary biliary cirrhosis: a double-blind, placebo-controlled trial on symptomatic patients. Aliment Pharmacol Therap 2001; 15(9): 1427–1434.

114. Kaplan MM, Cheng S, Price LL, and Bonis PA. A randomized controlled trial of colchicine plus ursodiol versus methotrexate plus ursodiol in primary biliary cirrhosis: ten-year results. Hepatology 2004; 39(4): 915–923.

115. Leuschner M, Maier K, Schlichting J, et al. Oral budesonide and ursodeoxycholic acid for treatment of primary biliary cirrhosis: results of a prospective double-blind trial. Gastroenterology 1999; 117(4): 918–925.

116. Rautiainen H, Kärkkäinen P, Karvonen AL, et al. Budesonide combined with UDCA to improve liver histology in primary biliary cirrhosis: a three-year randomized trial. Hepatology 2005; 41(4): 747–752.

117. Angulo P, Jorgensen RA, Keach JC, Dickson ER, Smith C, and Lindor KD. Oral budesonide in the treatment of patients with primary biliary cirrhosis with a suboptimal response to ursodeoxycholic acid. Hepatology 2000; 31(2): 318–323.

118. Angulo P, Patel T, Jorgensen R, Therneau TM, and Lindor KD. Silymarin in the treatment of patients with primary biliary cirrhosis with a suboptimal response to ursodeoxycholic acid. Hepatology 2000; 32(5): 897–900.

119. Talwalkar JA, Angulo P, Keach JC, Petz JL, Jorgensen RA, and Lindor KD. Mycophenolate mofetil for the treatment of primary biliary cirrhosis in patients with an incomplete response to ursodeoxycholic acid. J Clin Gastroenterol 2005; 39(2): 168–171.

120. Kurihara T, Niimi A, Maeda A, Shigemoto M, and Yamashita K. Bezafibrate in the treatment of primary biliary cirrhosis: comparison with ursodeoxycholic acid. Am J Gastroenterol 2000; 95(10): 2990–2992.

121. Nakamuta M, Enjoji M, Kotoh K, Shimohashi N, and Tanabe Y. Long-term fibrate treatment for PBC. J Gastroenterol 2005; 40(5): 546–547.

122. Nakai S, Masaki T, Kurokohchi K, Deguchi A, and Nishioka M. Combination therapy of bezafibrate and ursodeoxycholic acid in primary biliary cirrhosis: a preliminary study. Am J Gastroenterol 2000; 95(1): 326–327.

123. Ohira H, Sato Y, Ueno T, and Sata M. Fenofibrate treatment in patients with primary biliary cirrhosis. Am J Gastroenterol 2002; 97(8): 2147–2149.

124. Dohmen K, Mizuta T, Nakamuta M, Shimohashi N, Ishibashi H, and Yamamoto K. Fenofibrate for patients with asymptomatic primary biliary cirrhosis. World J Gastroenterol 2004; 10(6): 894–898.

125. Kanda T, Yokosuka O, Imazeki F, and Saisho H. Bezafibrate treatment: a new medical approach for PBC patients? J Gastroenterol 2003; 38(6): 573–578.

126. Sherlock S. Primary biliary cirrhosis (chronic intrahepatic obstructive jaundice). Gastroenterology 1959; 37: 574–586.

127. Fleming CR, Ludwig J, and Dickson ER. Asymptomatic primary biliary cirrhosis. Presentation, histology, and results with D-penicillamine. Mayo Clin Proc 1978; 53(9): 587–593.

128. Long RG, Scheuer PJ, and Sherlock S. Presentation and course of asymptomatic primary biliary cirrhosis. Gastroenterology 1977; 72(6): 1204–1207.

129. Roll J, Boyer JL, Barry D, and Klatskin G. The prognostic importance of clinical and histologic features in asymptomatic and symptomatic primary biliary cirrhosis. The N Engl J Med 1983; 308(1): 1–7.

130. Rydning A, Schrumpf E, Abdelnoor M, Elgjo K, and Jenssen E. Factors of prognostic importance in primary biliary cirrhosis. Scand J Gastroenterol 1989; 25: 119–126.

131. Metcalf JV, Mitchison HC, Palmer JM, Jones DEJ, Bassendine MF, and James OFW. Natural history of early primary biliary cirrhosis. Lancet 1996; 348: 1399–1402.

132. Shapiro J, Smith H, and Schaffner F. Serum bilirubin: a prognostic factor in primary biliary cirrhosis. Gut 1979; 20: 137–140.

133. Pares A and Rodes J. Natural history of primary biliary cirrhosis. Clin Liver Dis 2003; 7(4): 779–794.

134. Dickson ER, Grambsch PM, Fleming TR, Fisher LD, and Langworthy A. Prognosis in primary biliary cirrhosis: model for decision making. Hepatology 1989; 10(1): 1–7.

135. Kilmurry MR, Heathcote EJ, Cauch-Dudek K, et al. Is the Mayo model for predicting survival useful after the introduction of ursodeoxycholic acid treatment for primary biliary cirrhosis? Hepatology 1996; 23(5): 1148–1153.

136. Angulo P, Lindor KD, Therneau TM, et al. Utilization of the Mayo risk score in patients with primary biliary cirrhosis receiving ursodeoxycholic acid. Liver 1999; 19(2): 115–121.

137. Gores GJ, Wiesner RH, Dickson ER, Zinsmeister AR, Jorgensen RA, and Langworthy A. Prospective evaluation of esophageal varices in primary biliary cirrhosis. Gastroenterology 1989; 96: 1552–1559.

138. Levy C, Gomez JM, and Nelson D. Predictors of esophageal varices in patients with primary biliary cirrhosis. Hepatology 2005; 42(4(Suppl. 1)): 464-A.

139. Eastell R, Dickson ER, Hodgson SF, et al. Rates of vertebral bone loss before and after liver transplantation in women with primary biliary cirrhosis. Hepatology 1991; 14(2): 296–300.

140. Markus BH, Dickson ER, Grambsch PM, et al. Efficiency of liver transplantation in patients with primary biliary cirrhosis. N Engl J Med 1989; 320(26): 1709–1713.

141. Kim WR, Therneau TM, Poterucha JJ, et al. Optimal timing of liver transplantation for primary biliary cirrhosis. Hepatology 1998; 28(1): 33–38.

142. MacQuillan GC and Neuberger J. Liver transplantation for primary biliary cirrhosis. Clin Liver Dis 2003; 7(4): 941–956, ix.

143. Garcia RFL, Garcia CE, McMaster P, and Neuberger J. Transplantation for primary biliary cirrhosis: retrospective analysis of 400 patients in a single center. Hepatology 2001; 33(1): 22–27.

144. Tinmouth J, Tomlinson G, Heathcote EJ, and Lilly L. Benefit of transplantation in primary biliary cirrhosis between 1985–1997. Transplantation 2002; 73(2): 224–227.

145. Heathcote EJ, Stone J, Cauch-Dudek K, et al. Effect of pretransplantation ursodeoxycholic acid therapy on the outcome of liver transplantation in patients with primary biliary cirrhosis. Liver Transplant Surg 1999; 5(4): 269–274.

146. Christensen E, Gunson B, and Neuberger J. Optimal timing of liver transplantation for patients with primary biliary cirrhosis: use of prognostic modelling. J Hepatol 1999; 30(2): 285–292.

147. Kamath PS, Wiesner RH, Malinchoc M, et al. A model to predict survival in patients with end-stage liver disease. Hepatology 2001; 33(2): 464–470.

148. Jacob DA, Neumann UP, Bahra M, et al. Long-term follow-up after recurrence of primary biliary cirrhosis after liver transplantation in 100 patients. Clin Transplant 2006; 20(2): 211–220.

149. Levitsky J, Hart J, Cohen SM, and Te HS. The effect of immunosuppressive regimens on the recurrence of primary biliary cirrhosis after liver transplantation. Liver Transplant 2003; 9(7): 733–736.
150. Guy JE, Qian P, Lowell JA, and Peters MG. Recurrent primary biliary cirrhosis: peritransplant factors and ursodeoxycholic acid treatment post-liver transplant. Liver Transplant 2005; 11(10): 1252–1257.
151. Sanchez EQ, Levy MF, Goldstein RM, et al. The changing clinical presentation of recurrent primary biliary cirrhosis after liver transplantation. Transplantation 2003; 76(11): 1583–1588.
152. Neuberger J, Gunson B, Hubscher S, and Nightingale P. Immunosuppression affects the rate of recurrent primary biliary cirrhosis after liver transplantation. Liver Transplant 2004; 10(4): 488–491.
153. Neuberger J. Liver transplantation for primary biliary cirrhosis: indications and risk of recurrence. J Hepatol 2003; 39(2): 142–148.

4 Primary Sclerosing Cholangitis

Kelly Warren Burak

CONTENTS

Abstract

Primary sclerosing cholangitis is a chronic, progressive cholestatic liver disease characterized by fibrosis of the intra and extrahepatic bile ducts. It is frequently associated with inflammatory bowel disease. A typical patient with primary sclerosing cholangitis is a middle-aged male with ulcerative colitis with cholestatic liver biochemistries. The prevalence of the disease may be as high as 80-100 cases per million. Increasingly, MR cholangiography is being used instead of endoscopic retrograde cholangiopancreatography. Liver biopsy may be useful in helping establish the diagnosis, particularly if the patient is suspected of having the small duct variant of PSC in which the cholangiogram is normal. There is evidence that there may be a genetic predisposition based on the presence of HLA haplotypes and the association of ulcerative colitis is not yet defined. The condition is a progressive disease which slowly advances over time and may shorten life expectancy. The most severe problem that can develop is bile duct cancer. No effective medical therapy is yet available for the underlying disease. Ursodeoxycholic acid is perhaps the best studied, but data from long-term clinical trials demonstrating improved survival are not yet available. Liver transplantation is an option for patients with end-stage liver disease.

Key Words: Cholestasis; diagnosis; endoscopic retrograde cholangiography and pancreatography (ERCP); pathogenesis; natural history; ulcerative colitis; colorectal cancer; cholangiocarcinoma; therapy; ursodeoxycholic acid; liver transplantation.

From: *Clinical Gastroenterology: Cholestatic Liver Disease*
Edited by: K. D. Lindor and J. A. Talwalkar © Humana Press Inc., Totowa, NJ

Primary sclerosing cholangitis (PSC) is a chronic, progressive cholestatic liver disease characterized by fibrosis of the intra- and extrahepatic bile ducts *(1,2)*. PSC is frequently associated with inflammatory bowel disease (IBD) that involves the colon and an increased risk of colon cancer in these patients *(3)*. There is no established effective medical therapy for this condition and liver transplantation remains the only life-extending option for patients who develop complications of cirrhosis. Cholangiocarcinoma (CCA) is the most feared complication of PSC, in that it carries a poor prognosis and usually precludes patients from transplantation. This chapter will review the diagnosis, pathogenesis, natural history, and malignancy risk of PSC and will review treatment options which have been investigated for this condition.

1. DIAGNOSIS

The typical patient with PSC is a middle-aged male with underlying ulcerative colitis (UC) who has elevation of cholestatic liver tests (alkaline phosphatase) with or without symptoms of cholestasis (jaundice, pruritus, and fatigue). The male to female ratio of PSC is approximately 2:1, and although it can present from early childhood to late adulthood, the median onset of the disease is approximately 40 years *(1,4)*. More than two-thirds of cases are associated with IBD, and it can occur in association with both UC and Crohn's disease (CD) that involves the colon. The association with IBD ranges from a low of 21% in Japan *(5)* to 82% in a study from the European Union *(4)*. A population-based study from Norway found an incidence of 1.3 and a prevalence of 8.1 cases per 100,000 *(6)*. Investigators from different parts of the world have found that 2.4–4.0% of UC patients and 1.4–3.4% of CD patients will ultimately develop PSC *(4)*.

The gold standard for the diagnosis of PSC is the cholangiogram, which demonstrates focal strictures and areas of dilatation within the intra- and/or extrahepatic biliary system (Fig. 1A). Traditionally the cholangiogram has been performed by endoscopic retrograde cholangiography and pancreatography (ERCP) or percutaneous transhepatic cholangiography (PTC). However, as these procedures are invasive and associated with risks of pancreatitis and bleeding, they are now typically reserved for patients presenting with jaundice or cholangitis who are likely to require interventions such as balloon dilation or stenting dominant strictures. Noninvasive imaging of the biliary system with magnetic resonance cholangiography and pancreatography (MRCP) (Fig. 1B) has comparable diagnostic accuracy to ERCP *(7,8)* and is rapidly replacing ERCP in many centers for the diagnosis of PSC.

A B

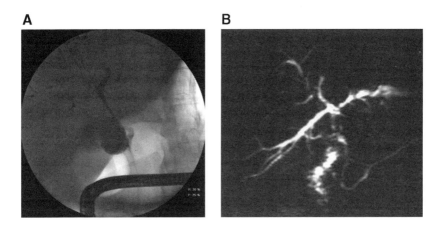

Fig. 1. (A) An ERCP of a 76-yr-old gentleman with unexplained cholestasis. He had no history of inflammatory bowel disease but the ERCP demonstrated focal area of stenosis, dilatation, and irregularity of the intrahepatic bile ducts consistent with PSC. **(B)** An MRCP of a 45-yr-old male with Crohn's colitis, who presented with cholestasis and pruritus, demonstrating beading within the bile ducts consistent with PSC.

The liver biopsy may help in establishing the diagnosis of PSC but is not essential in all patients *(9)*. The histologic findings of PSC are nonspecific and include bile duct inflammation or damage with corresponding ductopenia, cholestasis, and associated ductular proliferation *(10)*. Portal edema and mild periportal inflammation can also be seen. The classic finding of concentric fibrosis surrounding the bile ducts, the so-called onion-skin fibrosis (Fig. 2), is actually uncommon on liver biopsies from patients with PSC *(9)*. The histologic stage of fibrosis can provide prognostic value *(11)* and is included in many of the older models used to predict prognosis in PSC *(12–15)*. However, the new Mayo Risk Score (based on age, bilirubin, AST, variceal bleeding, and albumin) is able to predict prognosis without histologic stage *(16)*. Furthermore, sampling error is a significant problem in PSC and paired biopsies can yield very discrepant results *(17)*. A recent retrospective series from the Mayo Clinic concluded that liver biopsies are not necessary in all PSC patients because they rarely uncover unexpected findings that would lead to change in clinical management *(9)*.

A liver biopsy is necessary to diagnose the small duct variant of PSC, previously known as "pericholangitis," which accounts for approximately 5% of cases and generally has a better prognosis *(18–20)*. This diagnosis should only be made in patients with IBD

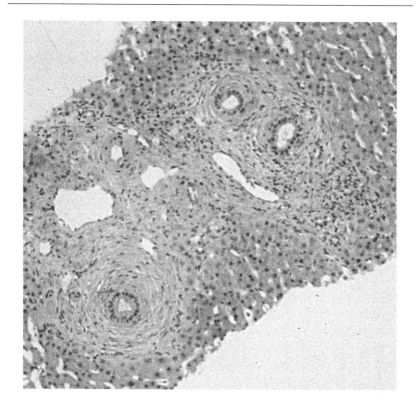

Fig. 2. A liver biopsy demonstrating "onion-skin" fibrosis around the bile ducts characteristic of PSC (H&E, mag. ×10).

who have changes in the liver biopsy consistent with PSC, but who have a normal cholangiogram and a negative antimitochondrial antibody (AMA) *(21)*. A biopsy may also be necessary when patients are suspected of having an overlap syndrome with autoimmune hepatitis (AIH) (discussed in Chapter 5) *(22,23)*.

2. PATHOGENESIS

Although the exact pathogenesis of PSC remains unknown, there have been many theories proposed to explain the development and progression of this chronic liver disease *(24)*. PSC likely develops in the setting of a complex interaction between a genetically susceptible host and the environment (colonic toxins, portal bacteria, or viral infections), with a possible role for autoimmunity, toxic bile acids, and ischemic injury *(25)*.

Evidence for genetic involvement in PSC includes disease occurrence within families and the association with several human leukocyte antigen (HLA) and non-HLA-associated genes *(24,25)*. A large study from Sweden found an increased prevalence of PSC among first-degree relatives (0.7%) and siblings (1.5%), representing nearly a 100-fold increased risk of developing PSC compared with the general population *(26)*. A large study from five European countries found PSC to be associated with several HLA class II haplotypes, with those homozygous for the DRB1*03, DQA1*0501, DQB1*02 haplotypes having the highest risk for PSC (RR=20, *P*<0.0001) *(27)*. However, this haplotype only accounted for 16% of 256 PSC patients in this study *(27)*.

Evidence for the role of autoimmunity in PSC includes its association with other immune-mediated conditions (most frequently UC), its HLA associations, and the presence of autoantibodies. Angulo and colleagues demonstrated the presence of autoantibodies in 97% of PSC patients with 81% having three or more autoantibodies *(28)*. The most common autoantibody is the peripheral antineutrophil nuclear antibody (p-ANNA), more commonly referred to as the p-ANCA (peripheral antineutrophil cytoplasmic antibody), which is seen in 33–88% of PSC patients *(29)*. The p-ANCA is nonspecific and can be seen in patients with AIH and primary biliary cirrhosis (PBC). It can provide supportive evidence for the diagnosis of PSC but the p-ANCA has no obvious association with disease activity or progression *(29)*. Less than half of PSC patients may have antinuclear antibodies (ANA) or antismooth muscle antibodies (ASMA) and the presence of AMAs is very rare *(28)*. Other abnormalities of the immune system have been demonstrated in patients with PSC including elevated immunoglobulin production, abnormalities in the complement system, and increased levels of circulating immune complexes *(25)*. Furthermore, the presence of autoantibodies may be more than an epiphenomenon and may in fact play a direct role in the pathogenesis of PSC. Fifteen years ago, Das and colleagues demonstrated antibodies directed against shared epitopes on biliary and colonic epithelium *(30)*. More recently, investigators from Sweden demonstrated antibiliary epithelial cell (anti-BEC) antibodies in 67% of patients with PSC *(31)*. These anti-BEC antibodies from PSC and PBC, but not AIH patients, induced interleukin 6 production from biliary epithelial cells (BEC); and antibody isolates from the serum of PSC, but not PBC and AIH patients, induced significantly increased expression of the cell adhesion molecule CD44 *(31)*.

Because of the strong association between colitis and PSC, it is hypothesized that colonic bacteria may be responsible for the immune stimulation seen in patients with PSC. Bacteria or bacterial products, which travel to the liver via the portal circulation, may stimulate the BEC or Kupffer cells which in turn may activate T cells *(24)*. The exact bacteria involved in this process have remained illusive, but *Chlamydia* and *Helicobacter* species have been suggested as putative candidates *(32,33)*. Others have postulated the role of viruses, including novel human beta-retroviruses, in the pathogenesis of cholestatic liver diseases *(34)*. The T-cell response in PSC is predominantly TH1 mediated and tumor necrosis factor alpha (TNFα) levels have been shown to be high in patients with PSC *(24)*. TNFα may result in further stimulation of the immune system, may worsen cholestasis, and may contribute to oxidative stress which hastens disease progression *(25)*. Adams and colleagues have postulated that memory T cells from an inflamed gut are rapidly recruited to the liver in response to hepatic inflammation *(35)*. Ischemic atrophy of BEC has been postulated to result in worsening cholestasis and biliary fibrosis, resulting in the accumulation of toxic bile acids which may further hasten disease progression *(25)*.

3. NATURAL HISTORY

PSC is a progressive condition which can result in symptoms related to cholestasis, recurrent episodes of ascending bacterial cholangitis, complications of portal hypertension (ascites, variceal bleeding, and encephalopathy), or the development of CCA. Pruritus, fever, and abdominal pain are the most common symptoms reported by patients with PSC *(36)*. Management of symptoms related to cholestasis (jaundice, pruritus, fatigue) is discussed elsewhere (Chapter 9). Patients who present with symptomatic liver disease are more likely to progress and have a significantly poorer prognosis compared to asymptomatic individuals (Fig. 3). The median survival free of death or liver transplantation in symptomatic individuals is approximately 8–9 years *(37)*. Although asymptomatic individuals have a better prognosis (approximately 75% survival at 7 years), their survival is significantly decreased compared to age-matched controls (Fig. 3) *(37)*. Whereas the development of complications of portal hypertension heralds the need to consider liver transplantation, the dreaded complication of CCA is typically felt to be a contraindication for transplantation and is associated with a very poor prognosis *(38)*. There has been a debate about transplanting PSC patients earlier to prevent CCA from occurring *(39,40)*.

Multiple models based on logistic regression have been developed to predict the natural history of PSC *(37)*. Most early models included

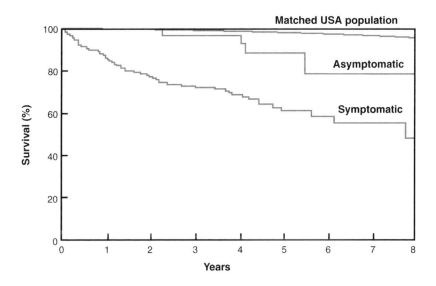

Fig. 3. The natural history of symptomatic and asymptomatic patients with PSC demonstrating decreased survival free of liver failure compared to age-matched controls (reproduced with permission from Ref. *[37]*).

histologic stage and age *(12–15)*, with many including bilirubin as a marker of disease severity *(12,13,15)* and others including splenomegaly *(13,14)*, hepatomegaly *(14)*, alkaline phosphatase *(14)*, or hemoglobin and IBD *(12)*. The new Mayo Clinic Risk Score no longer requires a liver biopsy (available at http://www.psc-literature.org/mrscalc.htm) and can stratify patients into low, medium or high risk of disease progression *(16)*. Others have suggested that the Child–Turcotte–Pugh (CTP) score is as good as the Mayo Clinic model in predicting outcomes in PSC patients *(41)*, although the Mayo Risk Score is likely better at predicting prognosis in patients with early disease *(42)*. The Model for End-stage Liver Disease (MELD), which is used to rank patients awaiting liver transplantation in the United States *(43)*, has not been specifically validated in a large population of PSC patients.

4. MALIGNANCY RISK IN PSC

The lifetime risk of CCA in patients with PSC is approximately 10% (range 4.8–36.4% in published studies) *(44)*. The rates are highest in series from tertiary care referral centers or liver transplant programs. A large population-based study found the risk of CCA in PSC to be approximately 13% *(45)*. Compared to the risk in the general population, the risk of CCA in PSC is dramatically elevated. A study of 161 PSC with 11.5 yr of median followup at the Mayo Clinic demonstrated a relative risk of CCA of 1560 (95% CI=780, 2793) compared to the SEER population database *(44)*. The prognosis for this malignancy is very poor with a median survival of only 6 mo *(46)*. Many patients are not candidates for surgical resection, because of extrahepatic spread or advanced liver disease at the time of diagnosis. In most centers the diagnosis of CCA is a contraindication to liver transplantation. However, investigators at the Mayo Clinic have reported acceptable patient survival and low recurrence rates of CCA using a protocol of chemotherapy, radiation, and staging laparotomy prior to transplantation in highly selected patients *(47,48)*. Small incidental CCA is often found in the explants of patients undergoing transplantation for PSC, and the survival of these patients is not significantly worse than for patients with PSC alone *(49)*.

Several studies have examined possible predictors for the development of CCA. More advanced disease as indicated by high bilirubin, higher Mayo Risk Scores, or complication of cirrhosis (variceal bleeding) have been found to predict CCA development in some studies *(15,44,50,51)*. The role of underlying IBD remains controversial, but patients with colorectal neoplasia do appear to carry an increased risk of CCA *(52)*. Smoking was associated with a risk of CCA in a Swedish study but this was not confirmed in a large study from the United States *(53,54)*. In the later study alcohol consumption was found to be a significant risk factor for the development of CCA *(54)*.

Various modalities are available to screen for CCA including serum tumor markers, ERCP-based tests, and more recently positron emission tomography (PET) scanning. These tests vary greatly in their expense, invasiveness, and availability. The CA19-9 is the most widely used noninvasive screening test for CCA. Its sensitivity and specificity vary widely depending on the cutoff point employed. A recent study from the Mayo Clinic found a CA19-9 cutoff of 129 U/ml provided reasonable diagnostic accuracy (sensitivity 79%, specificity 99%, positive predictive value 57%, and negative predictive value 99%) *(55)*. Furthermore, a change in CA19-9 overtime of 63 U/ml provided a sensitivity of 90%, specificity of 98%, and positive predictive value of 42% *(55)*. Therefore, patients with high or increasing CA19-9 levels should be viewed with suspicion for having malignancy. Unfortunately, only 2 out of 14 patients with CCA in this study were candidates for curative therapy, illustrating the limited impact of screening for CCA in this population *(55)*. In another study, 14 of 25 PSC patients with elevated CA19-9 were found to have a dominant stricture at ERCP and in 72% the CA19-9 fell following endoscopic dilation *(56)*. In this study, only three patients ultimately had CCA, illustrating the lack of specificity of an elevated CA19-9 *(56)*. Therefore, the role of tumor markers remains controversial, although many clinicians continue to order CA19-9 every 6 mo for screening for CCA.

When PSC patients present with jaundice or ascending cholangitis, ERCP is often used to investigate and manage strictures. All dominant strictures should be viewed as suspicious for CCA. Although associated with a high specificity, brushing with a sensitivity of ~50% or biopsies with a sensitivity of ~75% may still miss CCA *(57)*. Flow cytometry of bile and other techniques like digital image analysis may improve the diagnostic yield of ERCP-based tests but are not widely available *(58)*. The roles of cholangioscopy and intraductal ultrasound remain to be determined in PSC patients.

PET scanning has been investigated as a screening tool for CCA in patients with PSC. This test was initially suggested to have a good accuracy for the diagnosis of CCA with the added advantage of diagnosing distant metastases in many patients *(59,60)*. However, this test is limited by expense and availability and recent reports have suggested a limited role of PET to screen for CCA in PSC, because of a high false-positive rate when there is inflammation within the biliary system *(61)*.

The other malignancy which requires special attention in PSC patients is colorectal cancer (CRC) *(3)*. Patients with IBD carry an increased risk of CRC and dysplasia, which increases with the duration of colitis. Several studies have concluded there is an increased risk of CRC and colonic dysplasia in IBD patients with coexisting PSC compared to those without this liver disease *(45)*. A study from Sweden has suggested that the risk of CRC or dysplasia reaches 50% in PSC patients who have had coexisting colitis for more than 25-years duration (Fig. 4) *(52)*. It is recommended that patients with IBD who have coexisting PSC undergo increased surveillance colonoscopies to screen for dysplasia *(62)*. This is a cost-effective strategy, although there is recent evidence that these guidelines are not followed, even in tertiary referral centers *(63)*. The risk may be further increased in patients with colitis who have been transplanted for PSC *(64)*. These patients require increased surveillance with yearly colonoscopy after their liver transplant.

Interestingly, two studies have suggested that ursodeoxycholic acid (UDCA) may be of benefit in reducing risk of colorectal dysplasia or neoplasia in patients with PSC. In a cross-sectional survey from the

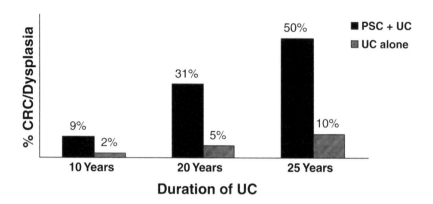

Fig. 4. The rates of dysplasia and colorectal cancer (CRC) in ulcerative colitis (UC) patients with and without PSC (adapted from Ref. *[52]*).

University of Washington, UDCA use was strongly associated with decreased prevalence of colonic dysplasia even after adjustment for sex, age at onset of colitis, duration of colitis, duration of sclerosing cholangitis, severity of liver disease, and sulfasalazine use with an adjusted odds ratio of 0.14 (95% CI=0.03, 0.64) *(65)*. Analysis of the patients in the Mayo Clinic randomized controlled trial of UDCA vs. placebo found a relative risk of 0.26 for developing colorectal dysplasia or cancer (95% CI=0.06, 0.92) in those PSC patients originally assigned to receive UDCA *(66)*. A more recent case–control study found no benefit of UDCA in preventing dysplasia or CRC, although mortality was lower in those receiving UDCA *(67)*. Although UDCA has not clearly been shown to delay disease progression in PSC patients, one could make an argument for its use in those patients with IBD as a potential chemo-preventative agent for CRC.

5. MANAGEMENT

Episodes of ascending cholangitis require not only broad-spectrum antibiotic coverage but also endoscopic therapy to diagnose and relieve biliary obstruction. Stenting is not clearly superior to balloon dilation alone for the management of dominant strictures *(68)*. Patients treated with the combination of endoscopic therapy and UDCA appear to have improved outcomes when compared to predicted survival from the Mayo Risk Score *(69)*. One retrospective surgical series found improved survival in patients whose dominant strictures were treated

Table 1
Therapies Without Proven Benefit in PSC

Bile acids	Immunosuppressive	Anti-TNF	Antifibrotic	Others
UDCA	Prednisone	Pentoxifylline	Colchicine	Nicotine
	Budesonide	Etanercept	Pirfenidone	Penicillamine
	Tacrolimus			Metronidazole
	Methotrexate			
	Mycophenolate mofetil			

Abbreviations: TNF, tumor necrosis factor; UDCA, ursodeoxycholic acid.

with surgical resection rather than with medical and endoscopic therapy, likely resulting from the development of five CCA in the later group *(70)*. However, biliary tract surgery is probably best avoided in patients with PSC. Recurrent episodes of ascending cholangitis can be managed by rotating oral antibiotics and may be an indication for liver transplantation.

To date there is no clearly effective medical therapy that has been shown to delay the progression of PSC (Table 1). UDCA has received the most attention as it has shown benefit in slowing the progression of PBC (discussed in Chapter 3). Standard doses of UDCA (13–15 mg/kg) were not better than placebo in delaying progression to treatment failure or need for liver transplantation in PSC *(71)*. It has been suggested that higher doses of UDCA may be beneficial *(72,73)*; however, a large multicenter European trial found no statistically significant beneficial effect of a UDCA (17–23 mg/kg) over placebo on survival or prevention of CCA *(74)*. Another large multicenter placebo-controlled trial of high-dose UDCA is underway in the United States.

Given the presumed role of autoimmunity in the pathogenesis of PSC, multiple immunosuppressive agents have been studied as potential treatments. Glucocorticoids do not have clear benefit in PSC *(75)*. A small randomized trial of prednisone vs. budesonide found improvement in ALP and pruritus in prednisone-treated patients *(76)*. However, another open-label study found budesonide to be associated with little clinical benefit and it significantly worsened osteoporosis in patients with PSC *(77)*. One-year therapy with tacrolimus resulted in improvements of ALP, ALT, AST, and bilirubin in 10 PSC patients *(78)*, but this agent has not been studied further in a large randomized clinical trial. An early report suggested that methotrexate (MTX) may improve symptoms in patients with PSC *(79)*; however, a subsequent open-label study found no benefit but increased toxicity when MTX was given with UDCA *(80)*. Furthermore, a 2-yr double-blind study found no evidence to support the use of MTX in PSC patients *(81)*. Mycophenolate mofetil has recently been found to have no benefit in an open-label study *(82)* and a small randomized clinical trial *(83)*.

Pilot studies of anti-TNFα agents, such as pentoxifylline *(84)* and etanercept, have yielded disappointing results. Antifibrotic agents such as pirfenidone *(85)* and colchicine *(86,87)* have proven ineffective. Because of an inverse relationship between smoking and risk of PSC, oral nicotine has been evaluated, but is poorly tolerated and without obvious benefit *(88)*. D-Penicillamine which modulates the immune system and chelates copper (which may be increased in cholestasis) was not beneficial *(89)*. A recent randomized clinical trial of UDCA+metronidazole vs. UDCA+placebo found an improvement in ALP and the new Mayo Risk Score in patients receiving the antibiotic; however, no benefit was seen in disease progression assessed by biopsy or ERCP *(90)*.

Liver transplantation (discussed further in Chapter 10) remains the only life-extending option for PSC patients with complications of end-stage liver disease. Subjects who do undergo liver transplantation can expect excellent survival rates, although transplantation for PSC is associated with higher rates of nonanastamotic strictures, rejection rates, colorectal neoplasia, and recurrence of the disease in approximately 20–40% of patients *(49,91)*.

REFERENCES

1. Angulo P and Lindor KD. Primary sclerosing cholangitis. Hepatology 1999; 30(1): 325–332.
2. Lee YM and Kaplan MM. Primary sclerosing cholangitis. N Engl J Med 1995; 332(14): 924–933.
3. Broome U and Bergquist A. Primary sclerosing cholangitis, inflammatory bowel disease and colon cancer. Semin Liver Dis 2006; 26(1): 31–41.
4. Schrumpf E and Boberg KM. Epidemiology of primary sclerosing cholangitis. Best Pract Res Clin Gastroenterol 2001; 15(4): 553–562.
5. Takikawa H and Manabe T. Primary sclerosing cholangitis in Japan—analysis of 192 cases. J Gastroenterol 1997; 32(1): 134–137.
6. Boberg KM, Aadland E, Jahnsen J, Raknerud N, Stiris M, and Bell H. Incidence and prevalence of primary biliary cirrhosis, primary sclerosing cholangitis and autoimmune hepatitis in a Norwegian population. Scand J Gastroenterol 1998; 33(1): 99–103.
7. Angulo P, Pearce DH, Johnson CD, et al. Magnetic resonance cholangiography in patients with biliary disease: its role in primary sclerosing cholangitis. J Hepatol 2000; 33(4): 520–527.

8. Berstad AE, Aabakken L, Smith, HJ, Aasen S, Boberg KM and Schrumpf E. Diagnostic accuracy of magnetic resonance and endoscopic retrograde cholangiography in primary sclerosing cholangitis. Clin Gastroenterol Hepatol 2006; 4(4): 514–520.
9. Burak KW, Angulo P and Lindor KD. Is there a role for liver biopsy in primary sclerosing cholangitis? Am J Gastroenterol 2003; 98(5): 1155–1158.
10. Ludwig J. Surgical pathology of the syndrome of primary sclerosing cholangitis. Am J Surg Pathol 1989; 13(Suppl 1): 43–49.
11. Scheuer PJ. Ludwig Symposium on biliary disorders—part II. Pathologic features and evolution of primary biliary cirrhosis and primary sclerosing cholangitis. Mayo Clin Proc 1998; 73(2): 179–183.
12. Wiesner RH, Grambsch PM, Dickson ER, et al. Primary sclerosing cholangitis: natural history, prognostic factors and survival analysis. Hepatology 1989; 10(4): 430–436.
13. Dickson ER, Murtaugh PA, Wiesner RH, et al. Primary sclerosing cholangitis: refinement and validation of survival models. Gastroenterology 1992; 103(6):1893–1901.
14. Farrant JM, Hayllar KM, Wilkinson ML, et al. Natural history and prognostic variables in primary sclerosing cholangitis. Gastroenterology 1991; 100(6): 1710–1717.
15. Broome U, Olsson, R, Loof L, et al. Natural history and prognostic factors in 305 Swedish patients with primary sclerosing cholangitis. Gut 1996; 38(4): 610–615.
16. Kim WR, Therneau TM, Wiesner RH, et al. A revised natural history model for primary sclerosing cholangitis. Mayo Clin Proc 2000; 75(7): 688–694.
17. Olsson R, Hagerstrand I, Broome U, et al. Sampling variability of percutaneous liver biopsy in primary sclerosing cholangitis. J Clin Pathol 1995; 48(10): 933–935.
18. Angulo P, Maor-Kendler Y, and Lindor KD. Small-duct primary sclerosing cholangitis, a long-term follow-up study. Hepatology 2002; 35(6): 1494–1500.
19. Bjornsson E, Boberg KM, Cullen S, et al. Patients with small duct primary sclerosing cholangitis have a favourable long term prognosis. Gut 2002; 51(5): 731–735.
20. Broome U, Glaumann H, Lindstom E, et al. Natural history and outcome in 32 Swedish patients with small duct primary sclerosing cholangitis (PSC). J Hepatol 2002; 36(5): 586–589.
21. Kim WR, Ludwig J, and Lindor KD. Variant forms of cholestatic diseases involving small bile ducts in adults. Am J Gastroenterol 2000; 95(5): 1130–1138.
22. Boberg KM, Fausa O, Haaland T, et al. Features of autoimmune hepatitis in primary sclerosing cholangitis: an evaluation of 114 primary sclerosing cholangitis patients according to a scoring system for the diagnosis of autoimmune hepatitis. Hepatology 1996; 23(6): 1369–1376.
23. Kaya M, Angulo P, and Lindor KD. Overlap of autoimmune hepatitis and primary sclerosing cholangitis: an evaluation of a modified scoring system. J Hepatol 2000; 33(4): 537–542.
24. Aoki CA, Bowlus CL and Gershwin ME. The immunobiology of primary sclerosing cholangitis. Autoimmun Rev 2005; 4(3): 137–143.
25. Cullen S and Chapman R. Aetiopathogenesis of primary sclerosing cholangitis. Best Pract Res Clin Gastroenterol 2001; 15(4): 577–589.
26. Bergquist A, Lindberg G, Saarinen S, and Broome U. Increased prevalence of primary sclerosing cholangitis among first-degree relatives. J Hepatol 2005; 42(2): 252–256.

27. Spurkland A, Saarinen S, Boberg KM, et al. HLA class II haplotypes in primary sclerosing cholangitis patients from five European populations. Tissue Antigens 1999; 53(5): 459–469.

28. Angulo P, Peter JB, Gershwin ME, et al. Serum autoantibodies in patients with primary sclerosing cholangitis. J Hepatol 2000; 32(2): 182–187.

29. Terjung B, Worman HJ. Anti-neutrophil antibodies in primary sclerosing cholangitis. Best Pract Res Clin Gastroenterol 2001; 15(4): 629–642.

30. Das KM, Vecchi M, and Sakamaki S. A shared and unique epitope(s) on human colon, skin and biliary epithelium detected by a monoclonal antibody. Gastroenterology 1990; 98(2): 464–469.

31. Xu B, Broome U, Ericzon BG, and Sumitran-Holgersson S. High frequency of autoantibodies in patients with primary sclerosing cholangitis that bind biliary epithelial cells and induce expression of CD44 and production of interleukin 6. Gut 2002; 51(1): 120–127.

32. Ponsioen CY, Defoer J, Ten Kate FJ, et al. A survey of infectious agents as risk factors for primary sclerosing cholangitis, are Chlamydia species involved? Eur J Gastroenterol Hepatol 2002; 14(6): 641–648.

33. Nilsson HO, Taneera J, Castedal M, Glatz E, Olsson R, and Wadstrom T. Identification of Helicobacter pylori and other Helicobacter species by PCR, hybridization and partial DNA sequencing in human liver samples from patients with primary sclerosing cholangitis or primary biliary cirrhosis. J Clin Microbiol 2000; 38(3): 1072–1076.

34. Mason AL, Xu L, Guo L, et al. Detection of retroviral antibodies in primary biliary cirrhosis and other idiopathic biliary disorders. Lancet 1999; 351(9116): 1620–1624.

35. Grant AJ, Lalor PF, Salmi M, Jalkanen S, and Adams DH. Homing of mucosal lymphocytes to the liver in the pathogenesis of hepatic complications of inflammatory bowel disease. Lancet 2002; 359(9301): 150–157.

36. Olsson R, Broome U, Danielsson A, et al. Spontaneous course of symptoms in primary sclerosing cholangitis: relationships with biochemical and histological features. Hepatogastroenterology 1999; 46(25): 136–141.

37. Talwalkar JA and Lindor KD. Natural history and prognostic models in primary sclerosing cholangitis. Best Pract Res Clin Gastroenterol 2001; 15(4): 563–575.

38. Bergquist A and Broome U. Hepatobiliary and extra-hepatic malignancies in primary sclerosing cholangitis. Best Pract Res Clin Gastroenterol 2001; 15(4): 643–656.

39. Crippin JS. Motion—patients with primary sclerosing cholangitis should undergo early liver transplantation: arguments against the motion. Can J Gastroenterol 2002; 16(10): 700–702.

40. Lee YM. Motion—patients with primary sclerosing cholangitis should undergo early liver transplantation: arguments for the motion. Can J Gastroenterol 2002; 16(10): 697–699.

41. Shetty K, Rybicki L, and Carey WD. The Child–Pugh classification as a prognostic indicator for survival in primary sclerosing cholangitis. Hepatology 1997; 25(5): 1049–1053.

42. Kim WR, Poterucha JJ, Wiesner RH, et al. The relative role of the Child–Pugh classification and the Mayo natural history model in the assessment of survival in patients with primary sclerosing cholangitis. Hepatology 1999; 29(6): 1643–1648.

43. Wiesner R, Edwards E, Freeman R, et al. Model for end-stage liver disease (MELD) and allocation of donor livers. Gastroenterology 2003; 124(1): 91–96.

44. Burak K, Angulo P, Pasha TM, Egan K, Petz J, and Lindor KD. Incidence and risk factors for cholangiocarcinoma in primary sclerosing cholangitis. Am J Gastroenterol 2004; 99(3): 523–526.

45. Bergquist A, Ekbom A, Olsson R, et al. Hepatic and extrahepatic malignancies in primary sclerosing cholangitis. J Hepatol 2002; 36(3): 321–327.

46. Rosen CB, Nagorney DM, Wiesner RH, Coffey RJ, Jr, and LaRusso NF. Cholangiocarcinoma complicating primary sclerosing cholangitis. Ann Surg 1991; 213(1): 21–25.

47. Hassoun Z, Gores, GJ and Rosen CB. Preliminary experience with liver transplantation in selected patients with unresectable hilar cholangiocarcinoma. Surg Oncol Clin N Am 2002; 11(4): 909–921.

48. Kaya M, de Groen PC, Angulo P, et al. Treatment of cholangiocarcinoma complicating primary sclerosing cholangitis: the Mayo Clinic experience. Am J Gastroenterol 2001; 96(4): 1164–1169.

49. Wiesner RH. Liver transplantation for primary sclerosing cholangitis: timing, outcome, impact of inflammatory bowel disease and recurrence of disease. Best Pract Res Clin Gastroenterol 2001; 15(4): 667–680.

50. Schrumpf E, Abdelnoor M, Fausa O, Elgjo K, Jenssen E and Kolmannskog F. Risk factors in primary sclerosing cholangitis. J Hepatol 1994; 21(6): 1061–1066.

51. Nashan B, Schlitt HJ, Tusch G, et al. Biliary malignancies in primary sclerosing cholangitis: timing for liver transplantation. Hepatology 1996; 23(5): 1105–1111.

52. Broome U, Lofberg R, Veress B, and Eriksson LS. Primary sclerosing cholangitis and ulcerative colitis: evidence for increased neoplastic potential. Hepatology 1995; 22(5): 1404–1408.

53. Bergquist A, Glaumann H, Persson B, and Broome U. Risk factors and clinical presentation of hepatobiliary carcinoma in patients with primary sclerosing cholangitis: a case-control study. Hepatology 1998; 27(2): 311–316.

54. Chalasani N, Baluyut A, Ismail A, et al. Cholangiocarcinoma in patients with primary sclerosing cholangitis: a multicenter case-control study. Hepatology 2000; 31(1): 7–11.

55. Levy C, Lymp J, Angulo P, Gores GJ, Larusso N and Lindor KD. The value of serum CA 19-9 in predicting cholangiocarcinomas in patients with primary sclerosing cholangitis. Dig Dis Sci 2005; 50(9): 1734–1740.

56. Petersen-Benz C and Stiehl A. Impact of dominant stenoses on the serum level of the tumor marker CA19-9 in patients with primary sclerosing cholangitis. Z Gastroenterol 2005; 43(6): 587–590.

57. Rumalla A and Baron TH. Evaluation and endoscopic palliation of cholangiocarcinoma. Management of cholangiocarcinoma. Dig Dis 1999; 17(4): 194–200.

58. Rumalla A, Baron TH, Leontovich O, et al. Improved diagnostic yield of endoscopic biliary brush cytology by digital image analysis. Mayo Clin Proc 2001; 76(1): 29–33.

59. Keiding S, Hansen SB, Rasmussen HH, et al. Detection of cholangiocarcinoma in primary sclerosing cholangitis by positron emission tomography. Hepatology 1998; 28(3): 700–706.

60. Kluge R, Schmidt F, Caca K, et al. Positron emission tomography with [(18)F]fluoro-2-deoxy-D-glucose for diagnosis and staging of bile duct cancer. Hepatology 2001; 33(5): 1029–1035.

61. Fevery J, Buchel O, Nevens F, Verslype C, Stroobants S, and Van Steenbergen W. Positron emission tomography is not a reliable method for the early diagnosis of cholangiocarcinoma in patients with primary sclerosing cholangitis. J Hepatol 2005; 43(2): 358–360.

62. Lashner BA. Colorectal cancer surveillance for patients with inflammatory bowel disease. Gastrointest Endosc Clin N Am 2002; 12(1): 135–143, viii.

63. Kaplan GG, Heitman SJ, Hilsden RJ, et al. A population-based analysis of practices and costs of surveillance for colonic dysplasia in patients with primary sclerosing cholangitis and colitis. Inflamm Bowel Dis 2007; June 28 [Epub ahead of print].
64. Vera A, Gunson BK, Ussatoff V, et al. Colorectal cancer in patients with inflammatory bowel disease after liver transplantation for primary sclerosing cholangitis. Transplantation 2003; 75(12): 1983–1988.
65. Tung BY, Emond MJ, Haggitt RC, et al. Ursodiol use is associated with lower prevalence of colonic neoplasia in patients with ulcerative colitis and primary sclerosing cholangitis. Ann Intern Med 2001; 134(2): 89–95.
66. Pardi DS, Loftus EV, Jr, Kremers WK, Keach J, and Lindor KD. Ursodeoxycholic acid as a chemopreventive agent in patients with ulcerative colitis and primary sclerosing cholangitis. Gastroenterology 2003; 124(4): 889–893.
67. Wolf JM, Rybicki LA, and Lashner BA. The impact of ursodeoxycholic acid on cancer, dysplasia and mortality in ulcerative colitis patients with primary sclerosing cholangitis. Aliment Pharmacol Ther 2005; 22(9): 783–788.
68. Kaya M, Petersen BT, Angulo P, et al. Balloon dilation compared to stenting of dominant strictures in primary sclerosing cholangitis. Am J Gastroenterol 2001; 96(4): 1059–1066.
69. Stiehl A, Rudolph G, Kloters-Plachky P, Sauer P, and Walker S. Development of dominant bile duct stenoses in patients with primary sclerosing cholangitis treated with ursodeoxycholic acid: outcome after endoscopic treatment. J Hepatol 2002; 36(2): 151–156.
70. Ahrendt SA, Pitt HA, Kalloo AN, et al. Primary sclerosing cholangitis: resect, dilate, or transplant? Ann Surg 1998; 227(3): 412–423.
71. Lindor KD. Ursodiol for primary sclerosing cholangitis. Mayo primary sclerosing cholangitis-ursodeoxycholic acid study group. N Engl J Med 1997; 336(10): 691–695.
72. Harnois DM, Angulo P, Jorgensen RA, Larusso NF, and Lindor KD. High-dose ursodeoxycholic acid as a therapy for patients with primary sclerosing cholangitis. Am J Gastroenterol 2001; 96(5): 1558–1562.
73. Mitchell SA, Bansi DS, Hunt N, Von Bergmann K, Fleming KA, and Chapman RW. A preliminary trial of high-dose ursodeoxycholic acid in primary sclerosing cholangitis. Gastroenterology 2001; 121(4): 900–907.
74. Olsson R, Boberg KM, de Muckadell OS, et al. High-dose ursodeoxycholic acid in primary sclerosing cholangitis: a 5-year multicenter, randomized, controlled study. Gastroenterology 2005; 129(5): 1464–1472.
75. Chen W and Gluud C. Glucocorticosteroids for primary sclerosing cholangitis. Cochrane Database Syst Rev 2004; (3): CD004036.
76. van Hoogstraten HJ, Vleggaar FP, Boland GJ, et al. Budesonide or prednisone in combination with ursodeoxycholic acid in primary sclerosing cholangitis: a randomized double-blind pilot study. Belgian-Dutch PSC Study Group. Am J Gastroenterol 2000; 95(8): 2015–2022.
77. Angulo P, Batts KP, Jorgensen RA, LaRusso NA, and Lindor KD. Oral budesonide in the treatment of primary sclerosing cholangitis. Am J Gastroenterol 2000; 95(9): 2333–2337.
78. Van Thiel DH, Carroll P, Abu-Elmagd K, et al. Tacrolimus (FK 506), a treatment for primary sclerosing cholangitis: results of an open-label preliminary trial. Am J Gastroenterol 1995; 90(3): 455–459.
79. Knox TA and Kaplan MM. Treatment of primary sclerosing cholangitis with oral methotrexate. Am J Gastroenterol 1991; 86(5): 546–552.

80. Lindor KD, Jorgensen RA anderson ML, Gores GJ, Hofmann AF, and LaRusso NF. Ursodeoxycholic acid and methotrexate for primary sclerosing cholangitis: a pilot study. Am J Gastroenterol 1996; 91(3): 511–515.

81. Knox TA and Kaplan MM. A double-blind controlled trial of oral-pulse methotrexate therapy in the treatment of primary sclerosing cholangitis. Gastroenterology 1994; 106(2): 494–499.

82. Talwalkar JA, Angulo P, Keach JC, Petz JL, Jorgensen RA, and Lindor KD. Mycophenolate mofetil for the treatment of primary sclerosing cholangitis. Am J Gastroenterol 2005; 100(2): 308–312.

83. Sterling RK, Salvatori JJ, Luketic VA, et al. A prospective, randomized-controlled pilot study of ursodeoxycholic acid combined with mycophenolate mofetil in the treatment of primary sclerosing cholangitis. Aliment Pharmacol Ther 2004; 20(9): 943–949.

84. Bharucha AE, Jorgensen R, Lichtman SN, LaRusso NF, and Lindor KD. A pilot study of pentoxifylline for the treatment of primary sclerosing cholangitis. Am J Gastroenterol 2000; 95(9): 2338–2342.

85. Angulo P, MacCarty RL, Sylvestre PB, et al. Pirfenidone in the treatment of primary sclerosing cholangitis. Dig Dis Sci 2002; 47(1): 157–161.

86. Lindor KD, Wiesner RH, Colwell LJ, Steiner B, Beaver S, and LaRusso NF. The combination of prednisone and colchicine in patients with primary sclerosing cholangitis. Am J Gastroenterol 1991; 86(1): 57–61.

87. Olsson R, Broome U, Danielsson A, et al. Colchicine treatment of primary sclerosing cholangitis. Gastroenterology 1995; 108(4): 1199–1203.

88. Angulo P, Bharucha AE, Jorgensen RA, et al. Oral nicotine in treatment of primary sclerosing cholangitis, a pilot study. Dig Dis Sci 1999; 44(3): 602–607.

89. LaRusso NF, Wiesner RH, Ludwig J, MacCarty RL, Beaver SJ, and Zinsmeister AR. Prospective trial of penicillamine in primary sclerosing cholangitis. Gastroenterology 1988; 95(4): 1036–1042.

90. Farkkila M, Karvonen AL, Nurmi H, et al. Metronidazole and ursodeoxycholic acid for primary sclerosing cholangitis: a randomized placebo-controlled trial. Hepatology 2004; 40(6): 1379–1386.

91. Bjoro K, Brandsaeter B, Foss A, and Schrumpf E. Liver transplantation in primary sclerosing cholangitis. Semin Liver Dis 2006; 26(1): 69–79.

5 Overlap Syndromes with Autoimmune Hepatitis

Alastair D. Smith

CONTENTS

Abstract

Autoimmune hepatitis, or some features thereof, may co-exist with primary biliary cirrhosis and primary sclerosing cholangitis. However, definitions of what constitutes overlap syndrome are variable. Thus, the true prevalence of these entities is unknown, and the best management approach uncertain.

Key Words: Autoimmune hepatitis; primary biliary cirrhosis; primary sclerosing cholangitis; definitions; overlap syndrome; outcome.

1. INTRODUCTION

Patients with either of the chronic cholestatic disorders, primary biliary cirrhosis *(1)* (PBC) and primary sclerosing cholangitis *(2)* (PSC), may demonstrate clinical, laboratory, and/or histological features of autoimmune hepatitis (AIH) *(3–5)*. These include significant elevations of serum aminotransferase, immunoglobulin G, and total protein concentrations, additional circulating antibodies, e.g., antinuclear (ANA), smooth muscle (SMA), and liver kidney microsomal (LKMA), and intense plasma

From: *Clinical Gastroenterology: Cholestatic Liver Disease*
Edited by: K. D. Lindor and J. A. Talwalkar © Humana Press Inc., Totowa, NJ

cell-predominant interface inflammation (hepatitis) that is responsive to systemic immunosuppressive therapy. Such features may be present and evident to varying degrees. Thus, in some circumstances it appears that two distinct entities exist rather than one—this may be especially true when the features develop separately rather than coexist from the outset. In others, that evidence may be subtler and so the distinctions less obvious, thereby making definitions somewhat hazy and therapeutic management less clear. For example, portal tract expansion with lymphocytes and the occasional plasma cell, in some cases spilling over into the lobules, i.e., interface hepatitis, is both a recognized and acceptable feature in patients with PBC *(6,7)*. However, the same abnormality involving most or all of the portal triads might raise questions as to whether the patient had concomitant AIH.

Experts are undecided as to the most appropriate explanation(s) for the simultaneous existence of features of AIH with either PBC or PSC *(5,8,9)*. Is it that two separate autoimmune disorders are present (there is evidence to support this view, in that one autoimmune condition may occur with another in 5–10% of patients) or that despite a number of features in common, e.g., PBC and AIH, the patient has a condition which is distinct from either? A third potential explanation is that the features may represent the middle part of a continuum extending from classical AIH at one end to classical PBC or PSC at the other. Lastly, it appears that a more exaggerated inflammatory response among patients with PBC or PSC who possess the B8, DR3, DR4 haplotype, found commonly in AIH, may be possible. An alternative view of this latter suggestion is that the diagnostic limits of one disorder may include features of another disease(s), but without there being a true overlap syndrome *(1)*. The purpose of this chapter is to provide a frame of reference that is as unambiguous as possible, yet acknowledges the continuing uncertainties of definition without compromising fundamental treatment principles. In so doing this might highlight potentially fruitful areas for further clinical research.

2. NOMENCLATURE

One potential reason for continued difficulty of perception where the idiopathic cholestatic disorders interface with AIH and vice versa is that several different terms describing the clinico-pathological elements present have gained popularity and acceptance through the years, notably with respect to PBC and AIH. Each descriptor has aimed to be more accurate than others before them, yet by their very emergence and continued existence have added some degree of uncertainty to our understanding. For example, the term autoimmune cholangitis or cholangiopathy has been characterized and understood in different ways during the past 20 years. It has been employed to describe patients with PBC in every other respect yet who lacked antimitochondrial antibody (AMA), i.e., AMA-negative PBC *(10–13)*. Other investigators refined this definition and reserved its use for patients with a cholestatic syndrome who were AMA negative, but strongly ANA and SMA positive *(14,15)*. Third, it has been used to describe patients in whom the predominant clinical, immunological, and histologic features were those of AIH *(16)*. Most recently, it has been used to define patients who were believed to have neither PBC nor AIH: these patients were identified prospectively, demonstrated both cholestatic and hepatitic features but had very limited responses to either steroids or ursodeoxycholic acid (UDCA), respectively *(17)*. It is worth stating that much of the published literature regarding the coexistence of features of AIH and the idiopathic cholestatic disorders has arisen either from relatively small series or from retrospective analyses of prospectively accumulated clinico-pathological data, notably liver biopsy material in which one or other disorder predominated, e.g., PBC. Therefore, to what extent this fully represents the overall extent and the true variability of the diseases is unclear. Nonetheless, it forms the basis for much of this review.

3. PRIMARY BILIARY CIRRHOSIS
AND AUTOIMMUNE HEPATITIS

It is probably worth reminding ourselves that the diagnostic pillars of PBC *(18)*, i.e., cholestatic liver test abnormalities, elevated IgM concentration, positive AMA titer (>1:40), lymphocytic portal tract inflammation, and medium-sized bile duct injury with subsequent loss *(18)*, lack specificity for this condition when considered in isolation from one another. This is especially true of the liver tests and histological abnormalities *(19)* which may be quite variable from one portal area to another in early stages of the disease with not only the evidence of granulomatous inflammation often lacking, but also the presence or absence of AMA. For example, not all of the 29 patients with a positive AMA titer followed thereafter for 15 years developed all the clinical manifestations of PBC *(20)*. Moreover, a negative AMA result by immunofluorescence does not imply that the same result will be achieved when different methods of testing are employed, e.g., ELISA or an immunoblot assay where the target autoantigen of M2 antibodies, a recombinant form of PDC-E2, is used *(21)*. Several studies have demonstrated significant false negative rates for AMA by immunofluorescence albeit among different patient populations, using one or other of the above techniques *(14,22–27)*.

3.1. Autoimmune Cholangitis

It seems unlikely that consensus regarding the definition and implications of the term autoimmune cholangitis will be achieved. On the one hand some investigators are firmly of the mind that it amounts to no more than AMA-negative PBC, is not a distinct clinico-pathological entity and certainly not to be entertained as an overlap syndrome *(8)*. They cite lack of specificity for a negative AMA result by immunofluorescence, variability of features consistent with AIH among PBC patients who lack AMA, namely lower or normal IgM levels and higher IgG concentrations, respectively, and greater ANA and SMA positivity with or without different staining patterns, e.g., nuclear rim immunoreactivity to a 210-kDa glycoprotein. Lastly, neither the presence of other AMA types, e.g., M4 or M9 *(28)*, nor the consistent expression of antibodies to an isotype of carbonic anhydrase has been able to discriminate patients with autoimmune cholangitis from those with PBC reliably *(29–31)*. Conversely, other authors believe that patients with a clinical syndrome that is distinct from both 'classical' AIH and PBC by virtue of possessing features common to both disorders and demonstrating a limited response to prednisone and/or UDCA deserves the right to be codified differently *(17)*. However, the implications of this particular designation with respect to treatment outcome, rate of disease progression, and requirement for orthotopic liver transplantation (OLT) are unknown as yet. Two earlier studies reported no significant differences in response to treatment with UDCA or requirement for OLT among patients with PBC according to their AMA status *(15,32)*.

3.2. PBC–AIH Overlap Syndrome

Turning now to overlap of PBC with AIH, disagreement among experts exists here also. It may be easier to accept the validity of the term overlap syndrome where first a demonstration of either classical PBC or AIH is followed after an interval of months or years by compelling features of the other disorder—so long as the features of the first disorder persist to some degree; otherwise, the term sequential might be more appropriate. However, both the literature *(33–36)* and personal experience suggest that such instances are rare. Instead, it is more common for 'diagnostic' features of both conditions to be present to a greater degree simultaneously, and it is in these circumstances that making the correct assignment of overlap syndrome rather than variant may be genuinely difficult, not to say controversial. For example, does the presence of an AMA titer (>1:40) in a patient who has AIH alone in all other respects *(5)* and who demonstrates an appropriate response to corticosteroid therapy constitute an overlap syndrome and carry the same validity as the coexistence of serologic and histologic (where the adequacy of biopsy size, staining, and interpretation is crucial) features of both AIH and PBC?

To my mind this is the key: in order to justify use of the designation "overlap syndrome" what minimum set of criteria must be satisfied? In some of the studies referred to earlier, the criteria adopted for diagnosis of PBC–AIH overlap syndrome were different. Chazouillères and colleagues identified 12 out of 130 (9.2%) patients with PBC in whom they believed PBC–AIH overlap existed: in all but one the features occurred simultaneously *(33)*. For the diagnosis to be satisfied patients had to demonstrate at least two of the accepted criteria for both conditions, namely elevated alkaline phosphatase (ALP) at least two times the upper limit of the normal range, a positive AMA result, and liver biopsy specimen that demonstrated a florid duct lesion (PBC) (Figure 1); and for AIH, an elevated alanine aminotransferase (ALT) concentration at least five times the upper limit of the normal range, an IgG level at least twice the upper limit of the normal range *or* a positive SMA titer (>1:40), and a liver biopsy revealing moderate to severe periportal or periseptal lymphocyte interface hepatitis (Figures 2 and 3). The same set of diagnostic standards was adopted for inclusion in a more recent study by the same group, in which the authors identified 17 patients (8.9%) with simultaneous PBC–AIH overlap syndrome *(37)*. By contrast, Lohse et al selected 14 patients from a large number seen in their department over 20 years based on an increased ALT concentration or high titer of either ANA or SMA in conjunction with a positive AMA result *(34)*. To this group was then added a further six patients whose liver biopsy findings were neither clearly those of PBC on the one hand nor those of AIH on the other (the biopsy findings themselves were not described in the paper, nor was the total number of patients from which the 20 were selected quoted).

Since then, other investigators have applied both the original (Table 1) and the subsequent (Tables 2–4). International Autoimmune Hepatitis Group (IAHG) scoring systems to patients with a secure diagnosis of PBC in the hope of maintaining a consistent and objective diagnostic assessment of potential PBC–AIH overlap syndrome *(38,39)*. In one

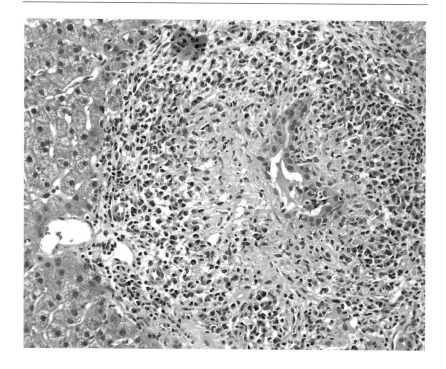

Fig. 1. Needle biopsy demonstrating florid duct injury typical of primary biliary cirrhosis with macrophage response surrounding the duct (Hematoxylin and eosin; x20).

case the difference was striking: under the original IAHG scoring system Talwalkar and colleagues documented 2.2% with definite AIH and 64% who met criteria for probable AIH in a large cohort of patients with PBC (137), whereas with the more recent modifications no patient had definite AIH, and a much reduced proportion (19%) had probable AIH *(40)*. The reasons for this are severalfold and may have more to say about some of the emphases in the revised scoring system, e.g., the weight assigned to the ALP:AST (aspartate aminotransferase) ratio, than about the true prevalence of the overlap syndrome.

Lastly, databases of the Canadian and Mayo Clinic multicenter, randomized controlled trials of UDCA in patients with AMA-positive PBC were re-examined to determine the frequency with which AIH was believed to co-exist. Like the French group, PBC patients in this study had to demonstrate at least two of the same three criteria

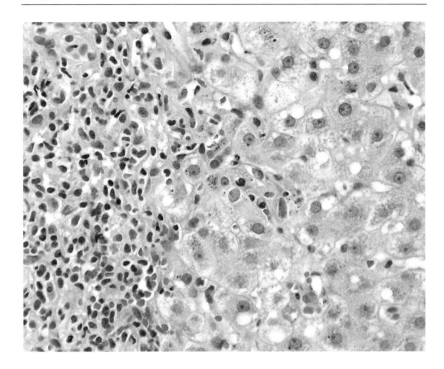

Fig. 2. Needle biopsy demonstrating irregularity of interface, infiltrated by plasma cells and lymphocytes; acidophilic necrosis in the adjacent lobule provides further evidence of injury consistent with autoimmune hepatitis (Hematoxylin and eosin; x20).

(see above) pointing strongly in favor of AIH. From a total of 331 patients with PBC, 16 (4.8%) were identified as fulfilling criteria for PBC-AIH overlap syndrome *(41)*.

A dedicated diagnostic scoring system has been developed and proposed in recent years to try and distinguish PBC from PBC–AIH overlap and other variant syndromes *(42,43)*. This underscores the importance of diagnostic accuracy between classical PBC and PBC–AIH overlap syndrome that goes beyond research purposes alone: both treatment strategies in these two settings and overall outcomes may vary.

3.3. Treatment of PBC–AIH Overlap Syndrome

Therapeutic management of PBC and AIH as individual entities is quite different. UDCA in doses of 13–15 mg/kg body weight per day

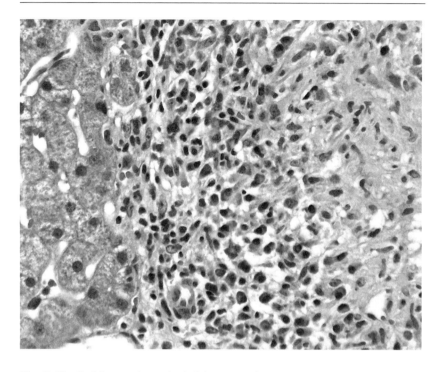

Fig. 3. Needle biopsy of portal triad (same as Figure 1) demonstrating infiltration of the interface by abundant plasma cells (Hematoxylin and eosin; x40).

is established treatment for PBC, resulting in reduction of ALP and IgM concentrations, improved histology, and longer duration between diagnosis and death or OLT. Conversely, systemic steroid therapy, which may be life-saving for patients with AIH, has no place in the management of PBC and may precipitate or exacerbate complications such as osteoporosis. Likewise, earlier trials demonstrated no clear benefit from azathioprine among patients with PBC (*6*).

As the reader has observed, given the differences in criteria used for definition of PBC–AIH overlap syndrome among investigators and that overall numbers of patients are few, it is not difficult to accept that randomized studies, the benchmark of therapeutic interventions, are unheard of in this setting. However, there are two retrospective analyses involving sufficient numbers of strictly defined patients that merit discussion and consideration. Joshi et al reviewed the outcome(s) of treatment that had been administered during a randomized placebo-controlled trial of UDCA for patients with PBC and concluded that those patients who met diagnostic criteria for PBC–AIH overlap syndrome fared no worse than those patients with PBC alone, with respect to both biochemical response and overall survival *(41)*. Furthermore, the degree of improvement in liver tests and serum IgM concentrations were similar in the two groups of patients, suggesting that UDCA was effective among patients with PBC–AIH overlap syndrome.

Conversely, Chazouillères et al examined the results of treatment using UDCA alone or UDCA in combination with prednisone and azathioprine or mycophenolate mofetil (IS therapy) for 17 patients with simultaneous PBC–AIH overlap syndrome (they used the same diagnostic criteria proposed in the 1998 report and employed by Joshi and colleagues in their study) *(37)*. Patients who started with UDCA alone but demonstrated an incomplete response were able to receive IS therapy since management was at the discretion of the supervising physician. They found that only 3/11 patients treated initially with UDCA alone were able to achieve and maintain biochemical remission defined as a reduction of ALT to less than two times the upper limit of the normal range and a serum IgG less than 16 g/l. The remaining eight (one patient declined for fear of side effects) required the addition of IS therapy to control disease and prevent progression of fibrosis. Among those patients managed using a combination of UDCA and IS therapy from the outset 66% achieved biochemical remission (see above), and none demonstrated progression of fibrosis. The authors concluded that for most patients with carefully defined PBC–AIH overlap syndrome, potential side effects notwithstanding, a combination of UDCA and steroid-based IS therapy will result in greatest long-term benefit.

Third, Gunsar and colleagues compared physician-directed management and outcomes for 23 patients with PBC to that of 20 patients with PBC-AIH overlap syndrome *(44)*. (Their criteria for defining PBC-AIH overlap syndrome were not identical to those of the two studies reported above). Nevertheless, two patients (9%) in the PBC group required addition of IS therapy (one was given azathioprine, and the other prednisone) because there was no improvement in ALP or other liver tests. By contrast, seven of the PBC-AIH group of patient required a combination (35%) required prednisone in combination with UDCA (four were given this at the onset of treatment and a further three after failure to respond to UDCA alone). A similar number of patients in either group died, or was lost to follow-up (2). The authors concluded that UDCA alone was appropriate first line therapy for patients with PBC-AIH overlap syndrome.

Table 1
Scoring System for Diagnosis of Autoimmune Hepatitis:
Minimum Required Parameters[a]

Parameters	Score
Gender	
Female	+2
Male	0
Serum biochemistry	
Ratio of elevation of serum alkaline phosphatase vs. aminotransferase	
>3.0	−2
<3.0	+2
Total serum globulin, γ-globulin or IgG	
Times upper normal limit	
>2.0	+3
1.5–2.0	+2
1.0–1.5	+1
<1.0	0
Autoantibodies (titers by immunofluorescence on rodent tissues)	
Adults	
ANA, SMA or LKM-1	
>1:80	+3
1:80	+2
1:40	+1
<1:40	0
Children	
ANA or LKM-1	
>1:20	+3
1:10 or 1:20	+2
<1:10	0
or SMA	
>1:20	+3
1:20	+2
<1:20	0
Antimitochondrial antibody	
Positive	−2
Negative	0
Viral markers	
IgM anti-HAV, HBsAg or IgM anti-HBc positive	−3
Anti-HCV positive by ELISA and/or RIBA	−2
Anti-HCV positive by PCR for HCV RNA	−3
Positive test indicating active infection with any other virus	−3

(*Continued*)

Table 1 (*Continued*)

Parameters	Score
Seronegative for all of the above	+3
Other etiological factors	
History of recent hepatotoxic drug usage or	
parenteral exposure to blood products	
Yes	−2
No	+1
Alcohol (average consumption)	
Male <35 gm/day; female <25 gm/day	+2
Male 35–50 gm/day; female 25–40 gm/day	0
Male 50–80 gm/day; female 40–60 gm/day	−2
Male >80 gm/day; female >60 gm/day	−1
Genetic factors	
Other autoimmune diseases in patient or first-degree relatives	+1

[a]**Interpretation of aggregate scores:** definite AIH, greater than 15 before treatment and greater than 17 after treatment; probable AIH, 10 to 15 before treatment and 12 to 17 after treatment.

Anti-HAV = hepatitis A virus antibody; *anti-HBc* = HBc antibody; *anti-HCV* = HCV antibody; *RIBA* = recombinant immunoblot assay; *PCR* = polymerase chain reaction.

Reproduced from HEPATOLOGY, Vol 18: 998–1005, Johnson PJ, McFarlane, IG.; "Meeting Report: International Autoimmune Hepatitis Group" © 1993 The American Association for the Study of Liver Diseases.

It is unclear whether the clinical outcome for patients with PBC–AIH overlap syndrome is significantly different from those with PBC alone. One recent report found that patients with PBC–AIH overlap syndrome (26/135) were more likely to demonstrate symptomatic manifestations of portal hypertension (ascites, gastrointestinal tract bleeding) than patients with PBC alone *(45)*. This argues in favor of a meticulous approach to diagnosis so that drug therapy and subsequent management might be tailored accordingly in the hope of preventing complications and disease progression. There is at least one report of the emergence of *de novo* autoimmune liver disease with PBC–AIH overlap features following OLT, involving a 56 year man who was grafted for non-alcoholic steatohepatitis *(46)*.

4. PRIMARY SCLEROSING CHOLANGITIS AND AUTOIMMUNE HEPATITIS

There are a number of reports, including single patients and small series *(47–66)*, documenting the occurrence of both PSC and AIH in adults, either simultaneously or in sequence. In the case of sequential

Table 2
Revised Scoring System for Diagnosis of Autoimmune Hepatitis

Parameters/Features	Score	Notes*
Female sex	+2	
ALP:AST (or ALT) ratio:		
<1.5	+2	1
1.5–3.0	0	
>3.0	−2	
Serum globulins *or* IgG above normal		
>2.0	+3	
1.5–2.0	+2	
1.0–1.5	+1	
<1.0	0	
ANA, SMA or LKM-I		
>1:80	+3	2
1:80	+2	
1:40	+1	
<1:40	0	
AMA positive	−4	
Hepatitis viral markers:		
Positive	−3	3
Negative	+3	
Drug history:		
Positive	−4	4
Negative	+1	
Average alcohol intake		
<25 g/day	+2	
>60 g/day	−2	
Liver histology:		
Interface hepatitis	+3	
Predominantly lymphoplasmacytic infiltrate	+1	
Rosetting of liver cells	+1	
None of the above	−5	
Biliary changes	−3	5
Other changes	−3	6
Other autoimmune disease(s)	+2	7
Optional additional parameters:		8
Seropositivity for other *defined* autoantibodies	+2	9
HLA DR3 or DR4	+1	10
Response to therapy:		
Complete	+2	11
Relapse	+3	

(*Continued*)

Table 2 (*Continued*)

Parameters/Features	Score	Notes*
Interpretation of aggregate scores:		
Pre-treatment:		
Definite AIH	>15	
Probable AIH	10–15	
Post-treatment:		
Definite AIH	>17	12
Probable AIH	12–17	

*See explanatory notes in Table 3. ALP = alkaline phosphatase; AST = aspartate aminotransferase; ALT = alanine aminotransferase; ANA = antinuclear antibodies; SMA = smooth muscle antibodies; LKM-l = type 1 liver-kidney microsomal antibodies.

diagnoses the more common order appears to be AIH *followed by* PSC. However, as one author observed, the absence of information from invasive cholangiographic studies at the time of diagnosis of AIH in some of these reports casts doubt as to whether the two disorders were indeed sequential, rather than simultaneous *(67)*. Whereas PBC–AIH overlap syndrome has been described in adults only, PSC and AIH may overlap in children. Indeed, a significant proportion of the published literature arises from studies in children and/or teenagers *(68–72)*. Moreover, results of these investigations suggest that the prevalence of PSC–AIH overlap syndrome is consistently greater among children (at least 27%, and as high as 49%) than in adults.

Since the diagnostic features of PSC and AIH are largely distinct from one another it would appear relatively straightforward to diagnose this overlap syndrome with confidence (PSC is characterized by multifocal intra- and/or extrahepatic biliary strictures, alternating with segmental bile duct dilatation, demonstrated at cholangiography: serum ALP is almost always elevated, the antineutrophil cytoplasmic antibody [ANCA] is almost always positive, and AMA is negative). However, analysis of the literature suggests that this is not necessarily the case. Among the case reports and small series, there appears fairly compelling evidence that features of PSC and AIH coexisted, irrespective of the pattern of onset and regardless of whether the diagnoses were simultaneous or sequential. Conversely, when large cohorts of patients with a secure diagnosis of PSC have been evaluated systematically using the IAHG scoring systems, reported rates of PSC–AIH overlap syndrome have ranged from 1.4% (definite AIH) to 53.8% at the other extreme when a modified version of the original IAHG scoring system was used *(54,57,59,60)*.

Table 3
Explanatory Notes for Table 2

1   The ALP:AST (or ALT) ratio relates to the decree of *elevation above upper normal limits* (unl) of these enzymes, i.e. = (IU/1 ALP÷unl ALP) ÷(IU/1 AST÷unl AST).

2   Titres determined by indirect immunofluorescence on rodent tissues or, for ANA, on HEp-2 cells. Lower titres (especially of LKM-1) are significant in children and should be scored at least +1.

3   Score for markers of hepatitis A, B and C viruses (i.e positive/negative for IgM anti-HAV, HBsAg, IgM anti-HBc, anti-HCV and HCV-RNA). If a viral aetiology is suspected despite seronegativity for these markers, tests for other potentially hepatotropic viruses such as CMV and EBV may be relevant.

4   History of recent or current use of known or suspected hepatotoxic drugs.

5   "Biliary changes" refers to bile duct changes typical of PBC or PSC (i.e. granulomatous cholangitis, or severe concentric periductal fibrosis, with ductopenia, established in an *adequate* biopsy specimen) and/or a substantial periportal ductular reaction (so-called marginal bile duct proliferation with a cholangiolitis) with copper/copper-associated protein accumulation.

6   Any other *prominent* feature or combination of features suggestive of a different aetiology.

7   Score for history of any other autoimmune disorder(s) in patient or first-degree relatives.

8   The additional points for other defined autoantibodies and HLA DR3 or DR4 (if results for these parameters are available) should be allocated *only* in patients who are seronegative lot ANA, SMA and LKM-1.

9   Other "defined" autoantibodies are those for which there are published data relating to methodology of detection and relevance to AIH. These include pANCA, anti-LC1, anti-SLA, anti-ASGPR, anti-LP and anti-sulfatide (see text).

10   HLA DR3 and DR4 are mainly of relevance to North European caucasoid and Japanese populations. One point may be allocated for other HLA Class II antigens for which there is published evidence of their association with AIH in other populations.

11   Assessment of response to therapy (as defined in Table 4) may be made at any time. Points should be added to those accrued for features *at initial presentation*.

12   Response and relapse as defined in Table 4.

The potential explanations for these observed differences are sever-alfold *(73)*. First, the mean ages of patients with PSC–AIH overlap syndrome in the study populations were different. Second, the scoring

Table 4
Definitions of Response to Therapy

Response	Definition
Complete	Either or both of the following: marked improvement of symptoms and return of serum AST or ALT, bilirubin and immunoglobulin values completely to normal within 1 year and sustained for at least a further 6 months on maintenance therapy, or a liver biopsy specimen at some time during this period showing at most minimal activity.
	or
	Either or both of the following: marked improvement of symptoms together with at least 50% improvement of all liver test results during the first month of treatment, with AST or ALT levels continuing to fall to less than twice the upper normal limit within 6 months during any reductions toward maintenance therapy, or a liver biopsy within 1 year showing only minimal activity.
Relapse	Either or both of the following: an increase in serum AST or ALT levels of greater than twice the upper normal limit or a liver biopsy showing active disease, with or without reappearance of symptoms, after a "complete" response as defined above.
	or
	Reappearance of symptoms of sufficient severity to require increased (or reintroduction of) immunosuppression, accompanied by any increase in serum AST or ALT levels, after a "complete" response as defined above.

Reprinted from JOURNAL OF HEPATOLOGY, Vol 31(5): 929–938, Alvarez F et al.; "International Autoimmune Hepatitis Group Report: Review of Criteria for Diagnosis of Autoimmune Hepatitis" © 1999 The European Association for the Study of the Liver.

systems used in the four studies were slightly different from one another. Boberg and colleagues used the original IAHG scoring system; Czaja employed a modified version thereof; van Buuren et al used the modified IAHG scoring system but did not specify detailed scores for each parameter. By contrast, colleagues from the Mayo Clinic established a diagnosis of AIH among patients with PSC using the modified scoring system exclusively. Although slightly confusing to the reader, the reality is that use of either the original or the subsequent IAHG scoring system in this setting makes little difference to the prevalence of 'definite' AIH, whereas the frequency of 'probable' AIH varied more considerably, being much reduced under the 1999 modified IAHG scoring system. (This was weighted strongly against biliary lesions, both in descriptive as well as in scoring terms.) Third, the findings may be subject to selection bias, geographical and/or genetic differences between Northern European and North American populations. Lastly, ALP may be normal in small numbers of patients with PSC, and ANCA may be present in up to 80% of patients with type 1 AIH alone *(74)*.

4.1. Treatment of PSC–AIH Overlap Syndrome

The differences in prevalence notwithstanding, it is clear from published reports that the distinction between PSC and PSC–AIH overlap syndrome is an important one to establish. Although corticosteroid therapy has no established place in management of PSC alone *(2)*, patients with simultaneous PSC and AIH or those who develop AIH following a diagnosis of PSC have demonstrated improvement in both symptoms and liver test abnormalities. The same cautions about steroid use among patients with PBC (see above) apply.

5. SUMMARY

Although there is considerable debate about how autoimmune overlap syndromes should be defined, and therefore their prevalence, their existence is not in doubt. Whether they reflect distinct clinical and histopathological entities or variants at the outer limits of 'classical' disease states remains the subject of considerable debate *(1)*. Nevertheless, published data indicate that the distinction is an important one to make, both with respect to therapeutic management and possibly disease outcome also.

REFERENCES

1. Czaja AJ. Overlap syndrome of primary biliary cirrhosis and autoimmune hepatitis: a foray across diagnostic boundaries (Editorial). J Hepatol 2006; 44: 251–252.
2. Levy C and Lindor KD. Primary sclerosing cholangitis: epidemiology, natural history, and prognosis (Review: 95 references). Semin. Liv Dis 2006; 26: 22–30.
3. Czaja AJ. and Freese DK. Diagnosis and treatment of autoimmune hepatitis (Review: 216 references). Hepatology 2002; 36: 479–497.
4. Czaja AJ, Bianchi FB, Carpenter HA, et al. Treatment challenges and investigational opportunities in autoimmune hepatitis. Hepatology 2005; 41: 207–215.
5. Krawitt EL. Autoimmune hepatitis (Review: 100 references). N Engl J Med. 2006; 354: 54–66.
6. Heathcote EJ. Management of primary biliary cirrhosis (Review: 105 references). Hepatology 2000; 31: 1005–1013.
7. Kaplan MM and Gershwin ME. Primary biliary cirrhosis (Review: 98 references). N Engl J Med 2005; 353 : 1261–1273.
8. Woodward J and Neuberger J. Autoimmune overlap syndromes (Review: 112 references). Hepatology 2001; 33: 994–1002.
9. Poupon R. Autoimmune overlapping syndromes (Review: 84 references). Clin. Liver Dis 2003; 7: 865–878.

10. Goodman ZD, McNally PR, Davis DR, and Ishak KG. Autoimmune cholangitis: a variant of primary biliary cirrhosis. Dig Dis Sci 1995; 40: 1232–1242.
11. Lacerda MA, Ludwig J, Dickson ER, Jorgensen RA, and Lindor KD. Antimitochondrial antibody-negative primary biliary cirrhosis. Am J Gastroenterol 1995; 90: 247–249.
12. Brunner G and Klinge O. A cholangitis with antinuclear antibodies (immunocholangitis) resembling chronic non-suppurative destructive cholangitis. Deutsche. Med Wochenschr 1987 ; 112: 1454–1458.
13. Taylor SL, Dean PJ, and Riely CA. Primary autoimmune cholangitis: an alternative to antimitochondrial antibody-negative primary biliary cirrhosis. Am J Surg Pathol 1994; 18: 91–99.
14. Michieletti P, Wanless IR, Katz A, et al. Antimitochondrial antibody negative primary biliary cirrhosis: a distinct syndrome of autoimmune cholangitis. Gut 1994; 35: 260–265.
15. Invernizzi P, Crosignani A, Battezzan PM, et al. Comparison of the clinical features and clinical course of antimitochondrial antibody positive and negative biliary cirrhosis. Hepatology 1997; 25: 1090–1095.
16. Ben-Ari Z, Dhillon AP, and Sherlock S. Autoimmune cholangiopathy: part of the spectrum of autoimmune chronic active hepatitis. Hepatology 1993; 18: 10–15.
17. Czaja AJ, Carpenter HA, Santrach PJ, and Moore SB. Autoimmune cholangitis within the spectrum of autoimmune liver disease. Hepatology 2000; 31: 1231–1238.
18. James OFW. Definition and epidemiology of primary biliary cirrhosis. In: Primary Biliary Cirrhosis (Neuberger, J., ed.) Eastbourne, West End Studios, 2000 pp. 53–59.
19. Weisner RH, LaRusso NF, Ludwig J, and Dickson ER. Comparison of the clinicopathological features of primary sclerosing cholangitis and primary biliary cirrhosis. Gastroenterology 1985; 88: 108–114.
20. Metcalf JV, Mitchison HC, Palmer JM, Jones DE, Bassendine MF, and James OFW. Natural history of early primary biliary cirrhosis. Lancet 1996; 348: 1399–1402.
21. Van de Water J, Cooper A, Surh CD, et al. Detection of autoantibodies to recombinant mitochondrial proteins in patients with primary biliary cirrhosis. N Engl J Med 1989; 320: 1377–1380.
22. Nakanuma Y, Harada K, Kaji K, et al. Clinicopathological study of primary biliary cirrhosis negative for antimitochondrial antibodies. Liver 1997; 17, 281–287.
23. Kitami N, Komada T, Ishii H, et al. Immunological study of anti-M2 in antimitochondrial antibody negative primary biliary cirrhosis. Intern Med 1995; 34: 496–501.
24. Kinoshita H, Omagari K, Whittingham S, et al. Autoimmune cholangitis and primary biliary cirrhosis—an autoimmune enigma. Liver 1999; 19: 122–128.
25. Nakajima M, Shimizu H, Miyazaki A, Watanabe S, Kitami N, and Sato N. Detection of IgA, IgM and IgG subclasses of anti-M2 antibody by immunoblotting in autoimmune cholangitis: is autoimmune cholangitis an early stage of primary biliary cirrhosis? J Gastroenterol 1999; 34: 607–612.
26. Tsuneyama K, van de Water J, van Thiel D, et al. Abnormal expression of PDC-E2 on the apical surface of biliary epithelial cells in patients with antimitochondrial antibody-negative primary biliary cirrhosis. Hepatology 1995; 22: 1440–1446.
27. Romero-Gómez M, Wichmann I, Crespo J, et al. Serum immunological profile in patients with chronic autoimmune cholestasis. Am J Gastroenterol 2004; 99: 2150–2157.

28. Davis PA, Leung P, Manns M, et al. M4 and M9 antibodies in the overlap syndrome of primary biliary cirrhosis and chronic active hepatitis: epitopes or epiphenomena? Hepatology 1992; 16: 1128–1136.
29. Gordon SC, Quattrociocchi-Longe TM, Khan BA, et al. Antibodies to carbonic anhydrase in patients with immune cholangiopathies. Gastroenterology 1995; 108: 1802–1809.
30. Invernizzi P, Battezzati PM, Crosignani A, et al. Antibody to carbonic anhydrase II is present in primary biliary cirrhosis irrespective of antimitochondrial antibody status. Clin Exp Immunol 1998; 114: 448–454.
31. Akisawa N, Nishimori I, Miyaji E, et al. The ability of carbonic anhydrase II antibody to distinguish autoimmune cholangitis from primary biliary cirrhosis in Japanese patients. J Gastroenterol 1999; 34: 366–371.
32. Kim WR, Poterucha JJ, Jorgensen RA, et al. Does antimitochondrial antibody status affect response to treatment in patients with primary biliary cirrhosis? Outcomes of ursodeoxycholic acid therapy and liver transplantation. Hepatology 1997; 26: 22–26.
33. Chazouillères O, Wendum D, Serfaty L, Montembault S, Rosmorduc O, and Poupon R. Primary biliary cirrhosis—autoimmune hepatitis overlap syndrome: clinical features and response to therapy. Hepatology 1998; 28: 296–301.
34. Lohse AW, zum Büschenfelde KH, Franz B, Kanzler S, and Gerken G. Characterization of the overlap syndrome of primary biliary cirrhosis (PBC) and autoimmune hepatitis: evidence for it being a hepatitic form of PBC in genetically susceptible individuals. Hepatology 1999; 29: 1078–1084.
35. Colombato LA, Alvarez F, Cote J, and Huet P-M. Autoimmune cholangiopathy: the result of consecutive primary biliary cirrhosis and autoimmune hepatitis? Gastroenterology 1994; 107: 1839–1843.
36. Horsmans Y, Piet A, Brenard R, Rahier J, and Geubel AP. Autoimmune chronic active hepatitis responsive to immunosuppressive therapy evolving into typical primary biliary cirrhosis syndrome: a case report. J Hepatol 1994; 21: 194–198.
37. Chazouillères O, Wendum D, Serfaty L, Rosmorduc O, and Poupon R. Long term outcome and response to therapy of primary biliary cirrhosis—autoimmune hepatitis overlap syndrome. J Hepatol 2006; 44: 400–406.
38. Johnson PJ and McFarlane IG. Meeting report: International Autoimmune Hepatitis Group. Hepatology 1993; 18: 998–1005.
39. Alvarez F, Berg PA, Bianchi FB, et al. International Autoimmune Hepatitis Group Report: review of criteria for diagnosis of autoimmune hepatitis. J Hepatol 1999; 31: 929–938.
40. Talwalkar JA, Keach JC, Angulo P, and Lindor KD. Overlap of autoimmune hepatitis and primary biliary cirrhosis: an evaluation of a modified scoring system. Am J Gastroenterol 2002; 97: 1191–1197.
41. Joshi S, Cauch-Dudek K, Wanless IR, et al. Primary biliary cirrhosis with additional features of autoimmune hepatitis: re°sponse to therapy with ursodeoxycholic acid. Hepatology 2002; 35: 409–413.
42. Yamamoto K, Terada R, Okamoto R, et al. A scoring system for primary biliary cirrhosis and its application for variant forms of autoimmune liver disease. J Gastroenterol 2003; 38: 52–59.
43. Gheorghe L, Iacob S, Gheorghe C, et al. Frequency and predictive factors for overlap syndrome between autoimmune hepatitis and primary cholestatic liver disease. Eur J Gastroenterol Hepatol 2004; 16: 585–592.

44. Günsar F, Akara US, Ersöz G, Karasu Z, Yüce G, and Batur Y. Clinical and biochemical features and therapy responses in primary biliary cirrhosis and primary biliary cirrhosis-autoimmune hepatitis overlap syndrome. Hepato-Gastroenterology 2002; 49: 1195–2000.

45. Silveira M, Talwalkar JA, and Lindor KD. Overlap of autoimmune hepatitis and primary biliary cirrhosis: long-term outcomes (Abstract). Gastroenterology 2006; 130 (Suppl 2), A-801.

46. Keaveny AP, Gordon FD, and Khettry U. Post-liver transplantation de novo hepatitis with overlap features. Pathology International 2005; 55: 660–664.

47. Minuk GY, Sutherland LR, Pappas SC, et al. Autoimmune chronic active hepatitis (lupoid hepatitis) and primary sclerosing cholangitis in two young adult females. Can J Gastroenterol 1988; 2: 22–27.

48. Rabinovitz M, Demetris AJ, Bou-Abboud CF, and Van Thiel DH. Simultaneous occurrence of primary sclerosing cholangitis and autoimmune chronic active hepatitis in a patient with ulcerative colitis. Dig Dis Sci 1992; 37: 1606–1611.

49. Perdigoto R, Carpenter HA, and Czaja AJ. Frequency and significance of chronic ulcerative colitis in severe corticosteroid-treated autoimmune hepatitis. J Hepatol 1992; 14: 325–331.

50. Lawrence SP, Sherman KE, Lawson JM, and Goodman ZD. A 39 year old man with chronic hepatitis. Semin Liver Dis 1994; 14: 97–105.

51. Wurbs D, Klein R, Terraccciano LM, Berg PA, and Bianchi LA. (1995) 28-year-old woman with a combined hepatitic/cholestatic syndrome. Hepatology 1995; 22: 1598–1605.

52. Gohlke F, Lohse AW, Dienes HP, et al. Evidence for an overlap syndrome of autoimmune hepatitis and primary sclerosing cholangitis. J Hepatol 1996; 24: 699–705.

53. Protzer U, Dienes HP, Bianchi L, et al. Post-infantile giant cell hepatitis in patients with primary sclerosing cholangitis and autoimmune hepatitis. Liver 1996; 16: 27–282.

54. Boberg KM, Fausa O, Haaland T, et al. Features of autoimmune hepatitis in primary sclerosing cholangitis: an evaluation of 114 primary sclerosing cholangitis patients to a scoring system for the diagnosis of autoimmune hepatitis. Hepatology 1996; 23: 1369–1376.

55. Luketic VAC, Gomez DA, Sanyal AJ, and Shiffman ML. An atypical presentation for primary sclerosing cholangitis. Dig Dis Sci 1997; 42: 2009–2016.

56. McNair ANB, Moloney M, Portmann BC, Williams R, and McFarlane IG. Autoimmune hepatitis overlapping with primary sclerosing cholangitis in five cases. Am J Gastroenterol 1998; 93: 777–784.

57. Czaja AJ. Frequency and nature of the variant syndromes of autoimmune liver disease. Hepatology 1998; 28: 360–365.

58. Koskinas J, Raptis I, Manika Z, and Hadziyannis S. Overlapping syndrome of autoimmune hepatitis and primary sclerosing cholangitis associated with pyoderma gangrenosum and ulcerative colitis. Eur J Gastroenterol Hepatol 1999; 11: 1421–1424.

59. van Buuren HR, van Hoogstraten HJF, Terkivatan T, Schalm SW, and Vleggaar FP. High prevalence of autoimmune hepatitis among patients with primary sclerosing cholangitis. J Hepatol 2000; 33: 543–548.

60. Kaya M, Angulo P, and Lindor KD. Overlap of autoimmune hepatitis and primary sclerosing cholangitis: an evaluation of a modified scoring system. J Hepatol 2000; 33: 537–542.

61. Griga T, Tromm A, Muller KM, and May B. Overlap syndrome between autoimmune hepatitis and primary sclerosing cholangitis in two cases. Eur J Gastroenterol Hepatol 2000; 12: 559–564.
62. Hatzis GS, Vassilou VA, and Delladetsima JK. Overlap syndrome of primary sclerosing cholangitis and autoimmune hepatitis. Eur J Gastroenterol Hepatol 2000; 13: 203–206.
63. Abdo AA, Bain VG, Kichian K, and Lee SS. Evolution of autoimmune hepatitis to primary sclerosing cholangitis: a sequential syndrome. Hepatology 2002; 36: 1393–1399.
64. Takiguchi J, Ohira H, and Shishido S. Autoimmune hepatitis overlapping with primary sclerosing cholangitis. Intern Med 2002; 41: 696–700.
65. Hong-Curtis J, Yeh MM, Jain D, and Lee JH. Rapid progression of autoimmune hepatitis in the background of primary sclerosing cholangitis. J Clin Gastroenterol 2004; 38: 906–909.
66. Floreani A, Rizzott ER Ferrara F, et al. Clinical course and outcome of autoimmune hepatitis/primary sclerosing cholangitis syndrome. Am J Gastroenterol 2005; 100: 1516–1522.
67. Rabinovitz M. Evolution of autoimmune hepatitis to primary sclerosing cholangitis (Letter). Hepatology 2003; 33: 946–947.
68. El-Shabrawi M, Wilkinson ML, Portmann BC, et al. Primary sclerosing cholangitis in childhood. Gastroenterology 1987; 92: 1226–1235.
69. Debray D, Pariente D, Urvoas E, Hadchouel M, and Bernard O. Sclerosing cholangitis in children. J Pediatr 1994; 124: 49–56.
70. Wilschanski M, Chait P, Wade JA, et al. Primary sclerosing cholangitis in 32 children: clinical, laboratory, and radiographic features, with survival analysis. Hepatology 1995; 22: 1415–1422.
71. Gregorio GV, Portmann B, Reid F, et al. Autoimmune hepatitis in childhood: a 20-year experience. Hepatology 1997; 25: 541–547.
72. Gregorio GV, Portmann B, Karani J, et al. Autoimmune hepatitis/ sclerosing cholangitis overlap syndrome in childhood: a 16-year prospective study. Hepatology 2001; 33: 544–553.
73. Chazouillères O. Diagnosis of primary sclerosing cholangitis—autoimmune hepatitis overlap syndrome: to score or not to score? (Editorial: 15 references). J Hepatol 2000; 33: 661–663.
74. Targan SR, Landers C, Vidrich A, and Czaja AJ. High-titer antineutrophil cytoplasmic antibodies in type-1 autoimmune hepatitis. Gastroenterology 1995; 108: 1159–1166.

6 Rare Causes of Cholestasis

Aaron J. Small and Konstantinos N. Lazaridis

CONTENTS

Abstract

Cholestasis is an important manifestation of a variety of liver diseases. Intrahepatic cholestasis can result from genetic defects of liver epithelial cells. Molecular studies in humans have provided insight into rare cholestatic syndromes such as Alagille syndrome, progressive familial intrahepatic cholestasis, benign recurrent intrahepatic cholestasis, and Aagenaes syndrome to name a few. Further characterization of these rare cholestatic disorders and the defective genes associated with them will aid in understanding hepatobiliary biology and other more common causes of intrahepatic cholestasis.

Key Words: Bile; cholestasis; transport.

1. INTRODUCTION

The term cholestasis, which literally means stagnation of bile in the liver, was first introduced by Popper and Schaffner *(1)*. Cholestasis can be classified into either extrahepatic or intrahepatic. Both result in failure of normal amounts of bile to reach the duodenum. Extrahepatic cholestasis is marked by an observed mechanical obstruction to the main bile ducts. In contrast, intrahepatic cholestasis occurs when there is an inherited or acquired defect of bile formation/transport within the liver epithelia (i.e., hepatocytes or biliary epithelia). Genetic and molecular

From: *Clinical Gastroenterology: Cholestatic Liver Disease*
Edited by: K. D. Lindor and J. A. Talwalkar © Humana Press Inc., Totowa, NJ

studies have identified several genes associated with intrahepatic cholestatic disorders. These disorders include Alagille syndrome (AGS), various forms of progressive familial intrahepatic cholestasis (PFIC), benign recurrent intrahepatic cholestasis, Aagenaes syndrome (AS), Northern American Indian cirrhosis (NAIC), and arthrogryposis, renal dysfunction, and cholestasis (ARC) syndrome.

This chapter elaborates on these rare causes of cholestasis. The majority of the aforementioned diseases appear to be Mendelian disorders, characterized usually by a variety of mutations in a single gene.

2. BILE FORMATION AND TRANSPORT

The hepatocytes produce "primary" or "hepatic" bile, which is subsequently delivered into the intrahepatic and then extrahepatic bile ducts before it arrives at the small intestine to serve its physiological functions. The intrahepatic bile ducts are lined by biliary epithelial cells, termed cholangiocytes that modify the composition of hepatic bile.

Primary bile is originated at the apical or canalicular domain of the hepatocyte with the contribution of transmembrane transporters. The majority of these molecules are ATP-binding cassette (ABC) transporters. Genetic defects of these hepatic transporters can cause rare inherited cholestatic diseases. However, other genes not directly interfering with the canalicular transport of bile likely contribute to the development of rare cholestatic syndromes.

3. RARE CHOLESTATIC SYNDROMES

3.1. Alagille Syndrome

AGS is an autosomal dominant disorder characterized by intrahepatic cholestasis and abnormalities of the heart, eye, and vertebrae, as well as a characteristic facial appearance. The prevalence of AGS has been reported to be approximately 1 per 100,000 births (2). Men and women are equally affected. AGS demonstrates low penetrance and high degree of expression variability (3–8,9).

Several reports of Alagille patients with deletions of chromosome 20p12 led to the incorrect thought that AGS is a contiguous gene deletion syndrome (10). However, fine mapping of the critical region directed two groups to simultaneously identify the gene JAG1 as the AGS gene (11,12). Indeed, both groups demonstrated that haplo-insufficiency of JAG1 results in AGS. JAG1 encodes a cell-surface protein that functions as a ligand for the Notch transmembrane receptor. The Notch pathway is active in many cells during development and serves to regulate cell fate decisions. The pathway was first studied in *Drosophila melanogaster* and found to be evolutionarily conserved. The multiple manifestations of AGS in humans suggest that JAG1 and Notch interactions are critical for normal embryogenesis of the heart, kidney, eye, face, skeleton, and other organs affected in this syndrome *(13,14)*.

To date, multiple mutations within the coding region of *JAG1* have been documented in patients with AGS. The majority of *JAG1* mutations in probands are new and not found in either parent *(15,16)*. Nonetheless, mutations can be present in 70% of patients who meet the clinical criteria for AGS *(17)*. Nearly half of these mutations are frameshift or nonsense mutations leading to premature truncation of the protein. The remaining mutations include gene deletions and missense mutations *(18)*. It is unclear as to whether missense mutations may cause milder variants of AGS or perhaps even single-organ abnormalities, though phenotypic differences between whole gene deletions and isolated point mutations have not been reported. Both copies of *JAG1* are necessary for normal embryogenesis in humans *(13,14,19)*. However, the mechanism by which mutated *JAG1* results in AGS remains unclear.

The clinical presentation of AGS is variable. Even within families, there is extreme variability in the severity of the disease, likely to be a result of other genetic and environmental modifying factors. Given the clinical variability and incomplete penetrance of the disorder, AGS often goes undiagnosed. Patients may present with progressive pruritus, cirrhosis, or liver failure. Still other individuals may lack or have few symptoms. Importantly, AGS is one of the more common etiologies of cholestasis in the neonatal period and must be differentiated from biliary atresia, which requires prompt surgical intervention. Affected patients generally develop symptoms within the first 3 mo of life. AGS may also present later in life as a chronic liver disease. Diagnosis is dependent on the characteristic liver histology showing bile duct paucity in addition to major extrahepatic findings including characteristic facies, cardiac murmurs, vertebral anomalies, and posterior embryotoxon. Conjugated hyperbilirubinemia in early infancy is the most common finding of AGS. Aminotransferases, particularly gamma glutamyl transferase (GGT), are modestly elevated. Bile acids may be as high as 100 times normal and serum cholesterol up to 1000–2000 mg/dl. Approximately 20% of patients develop progressive liver disease with 10–50% of these developing subsequent cirrhosis, liver synthetic dysfunction, or portal hypertension *(17)*. Despite these hepatic manifestations, the associated cardiac disease is most often responsible for the demise of the patients *(4,5,20)*.

There are currently no effective medical therapies for AGS. Supportive measures can be offered for nonspecific complications including pruritus. Ursodeoxycholic acid, rifampin, or antihistamines generally improve pruritus in patients with AGS. Ultimately, these patients may need orthotopic liver transplantation as the disease progresses toward end-stage liver disease. Children with severe pruritus but normal synthetic function may require biliary diversion as an alternative to liver transplantation *(21)*.

3.2. Progressive Familial Intrahepatic Cholestasis

PFIC represents a group of autosomal recessive disorders noted by the onset of cholestasis in infancy or early childhood that persists throughout life and often leads to liver cirrhosis within the first decade, unless treated *(22,23)*. Few patients have survived beyond the third decade of life. There are three types of PFIC (i.e., -1, -2, and -3) related to mutations in genes controlling the hepatocellular formation and transport of bile. Patients with PFIC-1 and PFIC-2 present with low serum GGT; patients with PFIC-3 have high serum GGT.

PFIC-1, also known as Byler's disease, was first described in Amish descendants of Jacob Byler *(24)*. PFIC-1 is characterized by low serum GGT, high serum bile salts, normal serum cholesterol, and low biliary chenodeoxycholic concentrations *(25,26)*. Positional cloning studies have mapped the mutation for PFIC-1 to the *FIC1* gene, which lies on a 19-cM region on chromosome 18q21–22 *(27–30)*. *FIC1* encodes a P-type ATPase (*ATP8B1*) involved in aminophospholipid transport from the outer to the inner leaflet of plasma membranes *(30)*. Expression of *FIC1* has been found in a number of tissues including the intestine, liver, biliary tract, pancreas, and kidney. Mutations in *FIC1*, in addition to causing PFIC-1, have also been linked to many cases of benign recurrent intrahepatic cholestasis (BRIC) and the cholestasis of Greenland Eskimos *(31,32)*.

The mechanism by which *ATP8B1* defects lead to PFIC-1 remains unknown. Dysfunctional bile acid excretion may be secondary to an altered lipid composition of the canalicular membrane of the hepatocyte. The farnesoid X receptor (FXR) may also play a role in the development of PFIC-1. Loss of *FIC1* alters the intestinal and hepatic bile acid transporter expression via diminished nuclear translocation of the FXR *(32)*. Dysregulation of bile acid transporters could potentially enhance ileal uptake and reduce canalicular secretion of bile salts to cause cholestasis.

Cases clinically similar to PFIC-1 were subsequently reported in non-Amish families in populations in the Middle East, Greenland, and Sweden. Mapping and linkage analysis in six consanguineous Middle

Eastern families identified the causative gene locus on chromosome 2q24 *(33,34)*. This disorder was designated PFIC-2. The cause of PFIC-2 is a gene that encodes for an ATP-dependent human bile salt export pump (BSEP, *ABCB11*) on the canalicular membrane of hepatocytes. *ABCB11* (i.e., BSEP) is an ABC transporter formerly known as sister of P-glycoprotein (SPGP) *(35)*. A variety of mutations (i.e., missense, nonsense, and deletional) have been identified in patients with PFIC-2 to cause the functional disturbances in bile salt excretion resulting in cholestasis *(36)*. In a study of 19 PFIC-2 patients, 10 lacked BSEP protein expression on the canalicular membrane *(37)*. As such, immunolocalization may provide a future means of diagnosing PFIC-2 in the appropriate clinical setting.

There are several clinical differences between PFIC-1 and PFIC-2. First, PFIC-1 patients present with a relapsing course of cholestatic symptoms in the early stages of the disease. Second, patients with PFIC-2 have a more rapidly progressive course to fibrosis than those with PFIC-1. Third, liver biopsies in PFIC-1 patients demonstrate a coarse granular bile and bland canalicular cholestasis. In contrast, PFIC-2 patients have amorphous or finely filamentous bile and neonatal hepatitis marked by inflammation with fibrosis and ductular proliferation *(27)*. Unlike Byler's disease, children with PFIC-2 do not have pancreatitis or watery diarrhea *(38,39)*.

PFIC-3 is characterized by high serum GGT and portal fibrosis with or without bile ductular proliferation *(40,41)*. Cholestasis occurs exceedingly early and can progress rapidly in these patients with the onset of cirrhosis and hepatic failure ranging from the neonatal period to early adulthood *(42,43)*. PFIC-3 is because of a mutation in the P-glycoprotein multidrug-resistance-3 (MDR-3) gene (i.e., *ABCB4*) on chromosome 7q21–36 *(41)*. As such, this disorder is also referred to as MDR-3 deficiency disease. MDR-3 is a primary active export pump that belongs to the family of ABC transporters and is expressed on the canalicular membrane of the hepatocyte. The molecule functions in the translocation of phosphatidylcholine across the canalicular membrane. Consequently, PFIC-3 patients lack MDR-3 on the canalicular domain of the hepatocyte and have a significant decrease (<15% of normal) in biliary phospholipid concentrations despite normal canalicular excretion of bile salts. Frame-shift and non-sense mutations of MDR-3 result in a truncated protein and seem to cause more severe disease than missense mutations which lead to a markedly reduced amount of MDR-3 mRNA *(43)*.

Similar to PFIC-2, MDR-3-deficient patients develop progressive liver disease characterized by portal inflammation, proliferation of bile ducts, and fibrosis. Interestingly, histology also shows small bile duct obstruction. This observation may come as a result of diminished biliary phospholipids, which can destabilize micelles and promote lithogenic bile with crystallized cholesterol *(44)*. Whether this instability of mixed micelles plays a role in the liver damage observed in patients with PFIC-3 is unclear. Injury to biliary epithelium may also result from direct and prolonged exposure to hydrophobic bile salts, which are normally offset by phospholipids in healthy individuals *(45)*.

Still further genetic heterogeneity in PFIC may exist. Several families with clinical and biochemical features consistent with PFIC-1 or -2 do not have linkage to either 18q (PFIC-1) or 2q (PFIC-2).

3.3. Benign Recurrent Intrahepatic Cholestasis

BRIC is characterized by intermittent attacks of jaundice and pruritus separated by symptom-free intervals *(46,47)*. Unlike PFIC, there is no permanent liver damage, no progression to cirrhosis, and no long-term complications of chronic liver disease *(48–50)*. Attacks consist of a 2- to 4-wk preicteric phase of malaise, anorexia, and pruritus, and an icteric phase lasting from 1 to 18 mo *(46,51)*. Attacks result in the characteristic cholestatic liver enzyme panel except that serum GGT remains low *(52)*. Surprisingly, liver biopsy shows no pathologic characteristics even during episodes. Clinical, laboratory, and histologic features of BRIC remain normal during the asymptomatic phase. Interestingly, BRIC has been mapped to the same 19-cM region of chromosome 18q21–22 as PFIC-1 *(28,53,54)*. In fact, Bull et al identified that mutations in *FIC1* (*ATP8B1*), the same gene affected in PFIC-1, can result in BRIC and that mutation type or location correlates with overall clinical severity *(30)*. BRIC also bears the same autosomal recessive inheritance as PFIC-1. For some patients with progressive cholestasis it would be difficult to distinguish whether they suffer from PFIC-1 or BRIC. As our methods to clinically identify and genetically characterize these patients improve, we will be in a better position to understand the pathogenesis of these syndromes.

Recently, various mutations in *ABCB11*, the same gene affected in PFIC-2, have been shown to be associated with a distinct type of BRIC, now classified as BRIC type 2 *(55)*. Of 11 patients with BRIC-2, none reported symptoms of pancreatitis, a known symptom of BRIC-1. BRIC-2 patients did, however, have a higher incidence of cholelithiasis *(55)*. Differences between BRIC type 1 and type 2 continue to be explored.

3.4. Dubin–Johnson Syndrome

Dubin–Johnson syndrome is a rare autosomal recessive liver disorder characterized by chronic conjugated hyperbilirubinemia, normal GGT and liver transaminases. The syndrome has also been linked to a defective bile canalicular membrane transporter for anion conjugates. Initial reports identified the transporter as canalicular multispecific organic anion transporter (cMOAT) encoded by the human gene MRP2 (*ABCC2*) located on chromosome 10q24 (*56,57*). This protein mediates ATP-dependent transport of a broad range of endogenous and xenobiotic compounds across the canalicular membrane of the hepatocyte. Defects in cMOAT may account for the impaired hepatobiliary transport of non-bile salt organic anions seen in patients with Dubin–Johnson syndrome. This is a rare syndrome with benign natural course. However, cases have been reported in which hepatocellular carcinoma was developed in the absence of other risk factors.

3.5. Crigler–Najjar Syndrome

Crigler–Najjar syndrome (CNS) is another rare genetic disorder resulting in chronic hyperbilirubinemia. Two types of CNS have been identified and recognized to be clinically distinct. Both are caused by an autosomal recessive defect in the *UGT1A1* gene complex with over 50 different mutations reported (*58*). This gene encodes for the enzyme uridine diphosphate (UDP) glycosyltransferase 1 family, polypeptide A1, known to conjugate bilirubin. In CNS type 1, there is complete absence of functional UGT1A1 so the unconjugated hyperbilirubinemia is severe. In contrast, some functional UGT1A1 activity is preserved in CNS type 2 (*59*). CNS type 1 and type 2 are further differentiated by their response to phenobarbitol. Phenobarbitol can significantly decrease serum bilirubin levels in CNS type 2 but has no effect on type 1. Interestingly, *UGT1A1* is also affected in the more common Gilberts syndrome, which presents with an even milder hyperbilirubinemia than CNS type 2. The varying degrees of hyperbilirubinemia in these disorders demonstrate the remarkable functional heterogeneity of mutations in the *UGT1A1* gene.

3.6. Cholestasis-Lymphedema Syndrome/Aagenaes Syndrome

AS is a very rare disorder representing the only known form of hereditary lymphedema associated with cholestasis. Initially reported in Norwegian families, this disorder has also been reported in children in other ethnic groups (*60–67*). AS demonstrates an autosomal recessive mode of inheritance, but a reported case of mother–child transmission suggests it may instead be autosomal dominant *(67)*. Although the mutation resulting in this familial cholestatic disorder remains unknown, the genetic locus, *LCS1*, has been mapped to chromosome 15q in a Norwegian kindred *(68)*. A second genetic locus, suggesting genetic heterogeneity of AS, may exist in other ethnic groups *(69)*. Patients with AS initially present with neonatal hepatitis, which later evolves into a chronic cholestatic condition and lymphatic disorder, particularly apparent in the lower limbs. It has been postulated that the pathogenesis of this condition is because of abnormal development of the hepatic lymphatics, though the underlying mechanism is not established. Initial cholestasis seems to resolve in early childhood, though recurrent bouts of cholestasis and lymphedema have been reported in adulthood *(62)*. Long-term liver damage or portal hypertension associated with this disease is rare.

3.7. Northern American Indian Cirrhosis

NAIC is a severe autosomal recessive intrahepatic cholestatic disease first described in Ojibway–Cree children from northwestern Quebec *(70)*. Retrospective studies suggest this disorder has a carrier frequency of 10% in the indigenous children of northwestern Quebec *(71)*. Patients with NAIC typically present with neonatal conjugated hyper-bilirubinemia and transient neonatal jaundice. Biliary cirrhosis and portal hypertension may occur in up to 90% of patients *(71)*. Serum amino-transferases, alkaline phosphatase, bile acids, cholesterol, and GGT all become elevated and persist despite resolution of neonatal jaundice. Light microscopy reveals giant cell hepatitis, biliary stasis, and neoductular proliferation. Notably, electron microscopy demonstrates widening of the pericanalicular microfilament cuff similar to changes seen in phalloidin intoxication *(70)*. Whether this marked accumulation of actin-containing microfilaments is because of dysfunctional contractile proteins or secondary to cholestatic injury is not known. As such, the cause of cholestasis could either be attributed to dysfunctional canalicular motility, a cholangiopathic phenomenon, or both. Some insight may be provided by the recent mapping of the genetic locus to chromosome 16q22. The defective gene was subsequently identified as a missense mutation in FLJ14728, conventionally called cirhin *(72)*. The encoded protein is preferentially expressed in embryonic liver, predicted to localize to mitochondria, and contains structural motifs frequently associated with molecular scaffolds. However, the function of cirhin and its role in NAIC pathogenesis remains unknown.

3.8. Arthrogyposis Multiplex Congenita, Renal Dysfunction, and Cholestasis Syndrome

ARC syndrome is an autosomal recessive multisystem disorder characterized by neurogenic arthrogryposis multiplex congenita, renal tubular dysfunction, and neonatal cholestasis marked by low GGT activity *(73–77)*. The neurogenic muscular atrophy is related to rarefaction of the anterior horn cells of the spinal cord. Affected infants generally die within the first year of life. Severe developmental delay, hypotonia, nerve deafness, poor feeding, microcephaly, and defects of the corpus callosum have been found in patients who survive infancy. Paucity of intrahepatic bile ducts and multinucleate transformation of hepatocytes have been reported as histologic features of ARC *(76,77)*. These patients may also develop renal tubular cell degeneration with nephrocalcinosis. Indeed, ARC is not associated with any chromosomal abnormalities or defects in mitochondrial or peroxisomal metabolism *(73)*. Instead, the disease has been mapped to a 7-cM interval on chromosome 15q26.1. Gissen et al recognized germline mutations in the gene VPS33B in 14 kindred with ARC. The encoded protein is a homolog of a vacuolar protein sorting gene found in yeast and an important regulator of vesicle-to-target SNARE-dependent membrane fusion *(78)*.

4. CONCLUSION

Owing to the advancement of genetic methodologies and molecular biology techniques we now have better understanding of the causes of rare cholestatic syndromes. These discoveries could form the foundation to elucidate the mechanisms of and devise novel therapies for less infrequent diseases of intrahepatic cholestasis.

REFERENCES

1. Sherlock S. Cholestasis: definition and classification of the major clinical forms. In: *Cholestasis* (Arias IM, McIntyre N, and Rodes J, eds), Elsevier Science, Amsterdam, 1994; pp. 3–19.
2. Danks DM, Campbell PE, Jack I, Rogers J, and Smith AL. Studies of the aetiology of neonatal hepatitis and biliary atresia. Arch Dis Child 1977; 52(5): 360–367.
3. Alagille D, Odievre M, Gautier M, and Dommergues JP. Hepatic ductular hypoplasia associated with characteristic facies, vertebral malformations, retarded physical, mental, and sexual development, and cardiac murmur. J Pediatr 1975; 86(1): 63–71.
4. Deprettere A, Portmann B, and Mowat AP. Syndromic paucity of the intrahepatic bile ducts: diagnostic difficulty; severe morbidity throughout early childhood. J Pediatr Gastroenterol Nutr 1987; 6(6): 865–871.

5. Emerick KM, Rand EB, Goldmuntz E, Krantz ID, Spinner NB, and Piccoli DA. Features of Alagille syndrome in 92 patients: frequency and relation to prognosis. Hepatology 1999; 29(3): 822–829.

6. LaBrecque DR, Mitros FA, Nathan RJ, Romanchuk KG, Judisch GF, and El-Khoury GH. Four generations of arteriohepatic dysplasia. Hepatology 1982; 2(4): 467–474.

7. Shulman SA, Hyams JS, Gunta R, Greenstein RM, and Cassidy SB. Arteriohepatic dysplasia (Alagille syndrome): extreme variability among affected family members. J Med Genet Am J Med Genet 1984; 19(2): 325–332.

8. Mueller RF, Pagon RA, Pepin MG, et al. Arteriohepatic dysplasia: phenotypic features and family studies. Clin Genet 1984; 25(4): 323–331.

9. Dhorne-Pollet S, Deleuze JF, Hadchouel M, and Bonaiti-Pellie C. Segregation analysis of Alagille syndrome. J Med Genet 1994; 31(6): 453–457.

10. Spinner NB, Rand EB, Fortina P, et al. Cytologically balanced t(2;20) in a two-generation family with alagille syndrome: cytogenetic and molecular studies. Am J Hum Genet 1994; 55(2): 238–243.

11. Li L, Krantz ID, Deng Y, et al. Alagille syndrome is caused by mutations in human Jagged1, which encodes a ligand for Notch1. Nat Genet 1997; 16(3): 243–251.

12. Oda T, Elkahloun AG, Pike BL, et al. Mutations in the human Jagged1 gene are responsible for Alagille syndrome. Nat Genet 1997; 16(3): 235–242.

13. Crosnier C, Attie-Bitach T, Encha-Razavi F, et al. JAGGED1 gene expression during human embryogenesis elucidates the wide phenotypic spectrum of Alagille syndrome. Hepatology 2000; 32(3): 574–581.

14. Jones EA, Clement-Jones M, and Wilson DI. JAGGED1 expression in human embryos: correlation with the Alagille syndrome phenotype. J Med Genet 2000; 37(9): 658–662.

15. Krantz ID, Colliton RP, Genin A, et al. Spectrum and frequency of jagged1 (JAG1) mutations in Alagille syndrome patients and their families. Am J Hum Genet 1998; 62(6): 1361–1369.

16. Crosnier C, Driancourt C, Raynaud N, et al. Mutations in JAGGED1 gene are predominantly sporadic in Alagille syndrome. Gastroenterology 1999; 116(5): 1141–1148.

17. Piccoli DA and Spinner NB. Alagille syndrome and the Jagged1 gene. Semin Liver Dis 2001; 21(4): 525–534.

18. Krantz ID, Piccoli DA, and Spinner NB. Clinical and molecular genetics of Alagille syndrome. Curr Opin Pediatr 1999; 11(6): 558–564.

19. Loomes KM, Underkoffler LA, Morabito J, et al. The expression of Jagged1 in the developing mammalian heart correlates with cardiovascular disease in Alagille syndrome. Hum Mol Genet 1999; 8(13): 2443–2449.

20. Alagille D, Estrada A, Hadchouel M, Gautier M, Odievre M, and Dommergues JP. Syndromic paucity of interlobular bile ducts (Alagille syndrome or arteriohepatic dysplasia): review of 80 cases. J Pediatr 1987; 110(2): 195–200.

21. Emerick KM and Whitington PF. Partial external biliary diversion for intractable pruritus and xanthomas in Alagille syndrome. Hepatology 2002; 35(6): 1501–1506.

22. Whitington PF, Freese DK, Alonso EM, Schwarzenberg SJ, and Sharp HL. Clinical and biochemical findings in progressive familial intrahepatic cholestasis. J Pediatr Gastroenterol Nutr 1994; 18(2): 134–141.

23. Jacquemin E. Progressive familial intrahepatic cholestasis. Genetic basis and treatment. Clin Liver Dis 2000; 4(4): 753–763.

24. Clayton RJ, Iber FL, Ruebner BH, and McKusick VA. Byler disease. Fatal familial intrahepatic cholestasis in an Amish kindred. Am J Dis Child 1969; 117(1): 112–124.

25. Tazawa Y, Yamada M, Nakagawa M, Konno T, and Tada K. Bile acid profiles in siblings with progressive intrahepatic cholestasis: absence of biliary chenodeoxy-cholate. J Pediatr Gastroenterol Nutr 1985; 4(1): 32–37.

26. Jacquemin E, Dumont M, Bernard O, Erlinger S, and Hadchouel M. Evidence for defective primary bile acid secretion in children with progressive familial intrahepatic cholestasis (Byler disease). Eur J Pediatr 1994; 153(6): 424–428.

27. Bull LN, Carlton VE, Stricker NL, et al. Genetic and morphological findings in progressive familial intrahepatic cholestasis (Byler disease [PFIC-1] and Byler syndrome): evidence for heterogeneity. Hepatology 1997; 26(1): 155–164.

28. Carlton VE, Knisely AS, and Freimer NB. Mapping of a locus for progressive familial intrahepatic cholestasis (Byler disease) to 18q21-q22, the benign recurrent intrahepatic cholestasis region. Hum Mol Genet 1995; 4(6): 1049–1053.

29. Bull LN, Juijn JA, Liao M, et al. Fine-resolution mapping by haplotype evaluation: the examples of PFIC1 and BRIC. Hum Genet 1999; 104(3): 241–248.

30. Bull LN, van Eijk MJ, Pawlikowska L, et al. A gene encoding a P-type ATPase mutated in two forms of hereditary cholestasis. Nat Genet 1998; 18(3): 219–224.

31. Klomp LW, Bull LN, Knisely AS, et al. A missense mutation in FIC1 is associated with greenland familial cholestasis. Hepatology 2000; 32(6): 1337–1341.

32. Chen F, Ananthanarayanan M, Emre S, et al. Progressive familial intrahepatic cholestasis, type 1, is associated with decreased farnesoid X receptor activity. Gastroenterology 2004; 126(3): 756–764.

33. Strautnieks SS, Kagalwalla AF, Tanner MS, et al. Identification of a locus for progressive familial intrahepatic cholestasis PFIC2 on chromosome 2q24. Am J Hum Genet 1997; 61(3): 630–633.

34. Strautnieks SS, Kagalwalla AF, Tanner MS, Gardiner RM, and Thompson RJ. Locus heterogeneity in progressive familial intrahepatic cholestasis. J Med Genet 1996; 33(10): 833–836.

35. Strautnieks SS, Bull LN, Knisely AS, et al. A gene encoding a liver-specific ABC transporter is mutated in progressive familial intrahepatic cholestasis. Nat Genet 1998; 20(3): 233–238.

36. Wang L, Soroka CJ, and Boyer JL. The role of bile salt export pump mutations in progressive familial intrahepatic cholestasis type II. J Clin Invest 2002; 110(7): 965–972.

37. Jansen PL, Strautnieks SS, Jacquemin E, et al. Hepatocanicular bile salt export pump deficiency in patients with progressive familial intrahepatic cholestasis. Gastroenterology 1999; 117(6): 1370–1379.

38. Winklhofer-Roob BM, Shmerling DH, Soler R, and Briner J. Progressive idiopathic cholestasis presenting with profuse watery diarrhoea and recurrent infections (Byler's disease). Acta Paediatr 1992; 81(8): 637–640.

39. Bourke B, Goggin N, Walsh D, Kennedy S, Setchell KD, and Drumm B. Byler-like familial cholestasis in an extended kindred. Arch Dis Child 1996; 75(3): 223–227.

40. Deleuze JF, Jacquemin E, Dubuisson C, et al. Defect of multidrug-resistance 3 gene expression in a subtype of progressive familial intrahepatic cholestasis. Hepatology 1996; 23(4): 904–908.

41. De Vree JM, Jacquemin E, Sturm E, et al. Mutations in the MDR3 gene cause progressive familial intrahepatic cholestasis. Proc Natl Acad Sci USA 1998; 95(1): 282–287.

42. Jacquemin E. Progressive familial intrahepatic cholestasis. J Gastroenterol Hepatol 1999; 14(6): 594–599.

43. Jacquemin E, De Vree JM, Cresteil D, et al. The wide spectrum of multidrug resistance 3 deficiency: from neonatal cholestasis to cirrhosis of adulthood. Gastroenterology 2001; 120(6): 1448–1458.

44. Elferink RP, Tytgat GN, and Groen AK. Hepatic canalicular membrane 1: The role of mdr2 P-glycoprotein in hepatobiliary lipid transport. FASEB J 1997; 11(1): 19–28.

45. Trauner M, Meier PJ, and Boyer JL. Molecular pathogenesis of cholestasis. N Engl J Med 1998; 339(17): 1217–1227.

46. Summerskill WH and Walshe JM. Benign recurrent intrahepatic "obstructive" jaundice. Lancet 1959; 2: 686–690.

47. Morton DH, Salen G, Batta AK, et al. Abnormal hepatic sinusoidal bile acid transport in an Amish kindred is not linked to FIC1 and is improved by ursodiol. Gastroenterology 2000; 119(1): 188–195.

48. Bijleveld CM, Vonk RJ, Kuipers F, Havinga R, and Fernandes J. Benign recurrent intrahepatic cholestasis: a long-term follow-up study of two patients. Hepatology 1989; 9(4): 532–537.

49. Nakamuta M, Sakamoto S, Miyata Y, Sato M, and Nawata H. Benign recurrent intrahepatic cholestasis: a long-term follow-up. Hepatogastroenterology 1994; 41(3): 287–289.

50. Putterman C, Keidar S, and Brook JG. Benign recurrent intrahepatic cholestasis— 25 years of follow-up. Postgrad Med J 1987; 63(738): 295–296.

51. Brenard R, Geubel AP, and Benhamou JP. Benign recurrent intrahepatic cholestasis. A report of 26 cases J Clin Gastroenterol 1989; 11(5): 546–551.

52. Lachaux A, Loras-Duclaux I, Bouvier R, Dumontet C, and Hermier M. Benign recurrent cholestasis with normal gamma-glutamyl-transpeptidase activity. J Pediatr 1992; 121(1): 78–80.

53. Houwen RH, Baharloo S, Blankenship K, et al. Genome screening by searching for shared segments: mapping a gene for benign recurrent intrahepatic cholestasis. Nat Genet 1994; 8(4): 380–386.

54. Sinke RJ, Carlton VE, Juijn JA, et al. Benign recurrent intrahepatic cholestasis (BRIC): evidence of genetic heterogeneity and delimitation of the BRIC locus to a 7-cM interval between D18S69 and D18S64. Hum Genet 1997; 100(3–4): 382–387.

55. van Mil SW, van der Woerd WL, van der Brugge G, et al. Benign recurrent intrahepatic cholestasis type 2 is caused by mutations in ABCB11. Gastroenterology 2004; 127(2): 379–384.

56. Kartenbeck J, Leuschner U, Mayer R, and Keppler D. Absence of the canalicular isoform of the MRP gene-encoded conjugate export pump from the hepatocytes in Dubin–Johnson syndrome. Hepatology 1996; 23(5): 1061–1066.

57. Paulusma CC, Kool M, Bosma PJ, et al. A mutation in the human canalicular multispecific organic anion transporter gene causes the Dubin–Johnson syndrome. Hepatology 1997; 25(6): 1539–1542.

58. Kadakol A, Ghosh SS, Sappal BS, Sharma G, Chowdhury JR, and Chowdhury NR. Genetic lesions of bilirubin uridine-diphosphoglucuronate glucuronosyltransferase (UGT1A1) causing Crigler–Najjar and Gilbert syndromes: correlation of genotype to phenotype. Hum Mutat 2000; 16(4): 297–306.

59. Seppen J, Bosma PJ, Goldhoorn BG, et al. Discrimination between Crigler–Najjar type I and II by expression of mutant bilirubin uridine diphosphate-glucuronosyltransferase. J Clin Invest 1994; 94(6): 2385–2391.

60. Aagenaes O, van der Hagen CB, and Refsum S. Hereditary recurrent intrahepatic cholestasis from birth. Arch Dis Child 1968; 43(232): 646–657.

61. Aagenaes O, Sigstad H, and Bjorn-Hansen R. Lymphoedema in hereditary recurrent cholestasis from birth. Arch Dis Child 1970; 45(243): 690–695.

62. Aagenaes O. Hereditary cholestasis with lymphoedema (Aagenaes syndrome, cholestasis-lymphoedema syndrome). New cases and follow-up from infancy to adult age. Scand J Gastroenterol 1998; 33(4): 335–345.

63. Aagenaes O. Hereditary recurrent cholestasis with lymphoedema—two new families. Acta Paediatr Scand 1974; 63(3): 465–471.

64. Sigstad H, Aagenaes O, Bjorn-Hansen RW, and Rootwelt K. Primary lymphoedema combined with hereditary recurrent intrahepatic cholestasis. Acta Med Scand 1970; 188(3): 213–219.

65. Vajro P, Romano A, Fontanello A, Oggero V, Vecchione R, and Shmerling DH. Aagenaes's syndrome in an Italian child. Acta Paediatr Scand 1984; 73(5): 695–696.

66. Nittono H and Unno A. Aagenaes syndrome. Ryoikibetsu Shokogun Shirizu 1995; (7): 521–522.

67. Morris AA, Sequeira JS, Malone M, Slaney SF, and Clayton PT. Parent–child transmission of infantile cholestasis with lymphoedema (Aagenaes syndrome). J Med Genet 1997; 34(10): 852–853.

68. Bull LN, Roche E, Song EJ, et al. Mapping of the locus for cholestasis-lymphedema syndrome (Aagenaes syndrome) to a 6.6-cM interval on chromosome 15q. Am J Hum Genet 2000; 67(4): 994–999.

69. Fruhwirth M, Janecke AR, Muller T, et al. Evidence for genetic heterogeneity in lymphedema-cholestasis syndrome. J Pediatr 2003; 142(4): 441–447.

70. Weber AM, Tuchweber B, Yousef I, et al. Severe familial cholestasis in North American Indian children: a clinical model of microfilament dysfunction? Gastroenterology 1981; 81(4): 653–662.

71. Drouin E, Russo P, Tuchweber B, Mitchell G. and Rasquin-Weber A. North American Indian cirrhosis in children: a review of 30 cases. J Pediatr Gastroenterol Nutr 2000; 31(4): 395–404.

72. Chagnon P, Michaud J, Mitchell G, et al. A missense mutation (R565W) in cirhin (FLJ14728) in North American Indian childhood cirrhosis. Am J Hum Genet 2002; 71(6): 1443–1449.

73. Nezelof C, Dupart MC, Jaubert F, and Eliachar E. A lethal familial syndrome associating arthrogryposis multiplex congenita, renal dysfunction, and a cholestatic and pigmentary liver disease. J Pediatr 1979; 94(2): 258–260.

74. Saraiva JM, Lemos C, Goncalves I, Carneiro F, and Mota HC. Arthrogryposis multiplex congenita with renal and hepatic abnormalities in a female infant. J Pediatr 1990; 117(5): 761–763.

75. Saraiva JM, Lemos C, Goncalves I, Mota HC, and Carneiro F. Arthrogryposis multiplex congenita with renal and hepatic abnormalities. Am J Med Genet 1992; 42(1): 140.

76. Horslen SP, Quarrell OW, and Tanner MS. Liver histology in the arthrogryposis multiplex congenita, renal dysfunction, and cholestasis (ARC) syndrome: report of three new cases and review. J Med Genet 1994; 31(1): 62–64.
77. Di Rocco M, Callea F, Pollice B, Faraci M, Campiani F, and Borrone C. Arthrogryposis, renal dysfunction and cholestasis syndrome: report of five patients from three Italian families. Eur J Pediatr 1995; 154(10): 835–839.
78. Gissen P, Johnson CA, Morgan NV, et al. Mutations in VPS33B, encoding a regulator of SNARE-dependent membrane fusion, cause arthrogryposis-renal dysfunction-cholestasis (ARC) syndrome. Nat Genet 2004; 36(4): 400–404.

7 Cholestatic Variants of Viral Disease and Alcohol

Sakib Khalid and Jeffrey S. Crippin

CONTENTS

INTRODUCTION
CHOLESTATIC VARIANT OF VIRAL HEPATITIS
CHOLESTATIC VARIANT OF ALCOHOLIC LIVER DISEASE
SUMMARY
REFERENCES

Abstract

Hepatitis of any etiology routinely presents with elevated transaminases. However, the presence of cholestasis should not necessarily rule out the presence of viral or alcoholic hepatitis. Hepatotropic viruses, such as hepatitis A, B, C, and E, can present with an elevated alkaline phosphatase and hyperbilirubinemia. Cytomegalovirus and Epstein–Barr virus infections may also present in this manner. Alcoholic hepatitis, often defined by an AST/ALT ratio of 2–3:1, can have cholestatic characteristics, as well. A careful clinical history, viral serologies, and, in some cases, a liver biopsy can clarify these disease states.

Key Words: Cholestasis; hepatitis A; hepatitis B; hepatitis C; hepatitis E; fibrosing cholestatic hepatitis; cytomegalovirus; Epstein–Barr virus; immunosuppression; liver transplantation; kidney transplantation; alcoholic hepatitis.

1. INTRODUCTION

Patients with viral hepatitis or alcoholic hepatitis routinely present with transaminase elevations. Those afflicted with one of the viral hepatitides may have transaminase levels in the thousands, whereas those with alcoholic hepatitis have an AST to ALT ratio of 2–3:1. However, cholestasis may occur with either of these disease states.

From: *Clinical Gastroenterology: Cholestatic Liver Disease*
Edited by: K. D. Lindor and J. A. Talwalkar © Humana Press Inc., Totowa, NJ

Recognizing this variant may be the key to making a timely diagnosis and instituting appropriate therapy.

2. CHOLESTATIC VARIANT OF VIRAL HEPATITIS

Viral hepatitis routinely presents with markedly elevated transminases, with cholestasis a less common finding. Among hepatotropic viruses, hepatitis A, B, C, and E can present with cholestasis. Cytomegalovirus (CMV) and Epstein–Barr virus (EBV) have also been associated with cholestatic changes. Cholestatic variants of hepatitis A and E affect immunocompetent hosts, whereas those of hepatitis B, C, CMV, and EBV primarily occur in immunocompromised hosts (1). The cholestatic variant of viral hepatitis was first reported in 1937 by Eppinger, who described a syndrome characterized by prolonged jaundice and cholestasis (2). Subsequently, cases of cholestatic hepatitis were described, presenting with fever, intense pruritus, prolonged jaundice, and an elevated alkaline phosphatase (3–6). Owing to the lack of serologic testing at that time, the exact virus responsible for this variant was unclear (7).

2.1. Hepatitis A

Hepatitis A causes an acute hepatitis, often presenting as an anicteric and subclinical illness. Adults are more likely to present with an icteric hepatitis. The disease resolves without sequelae in most patients. In rare cases, fulminant hepatitis may develop. Other atypical manifestations include a protracted hepatitis, relapsing hepatitis, and prolonged cholestasis (8–10).

Cholestatic hepatitis A was first described in 1982 when hepatitis A was found to be associated with cholestatic laboratory abnormalities (11). Another study described six patients with pruritus, fever, anorexia, diarrhea, and weight loss, subsequently found to have acute hepatitis A based on the presence of IgM antibody to the hepatitis A virus (12). Serum bilirubin levels peaked at greater than 10 g/dl, and the clinical course lasted at least 12 wk. In this study, five out of the six patients required hospitalization for supportive care; however, all patients recovered completely without sequelae.

The prevalence of cholestatic hepatitis A is quite low. One study found prolonged cholestasis in 1–10% of cases (9,13–17). Patients with cholestatic hepatitis A present with significant jaundice, pruritus, weight loss, diarrhea, and fever persisting for several weeks after the initial presentation or with a relapsing hepatitis (8,12). Rare associations with the cholestatic variant of hepatitis A include pancreatitis in children *(18)*, cutaneous vasculitis and cryoglobulinemia *(19)*, and toxic epidermal necrolysis *(20)*. In rare instances, acute renal insufficiency is associated with cholestatic hepatitis A. Acute tubular necrosis, interstitial nephritis, or glomerulonephritis have been seen *(21–27)*. Thirty-two patients with renal insufficiency associated with cholestatic hepatitis A have been described. In 29 of these patients, renal function returned to normal, only partial recovery of renal function was found in another, and 3 patients died resulting from other complications. In 19 (66%) patients, dialysis was necessary, whereas 2 required plasmapheresis. In the remaining 11 patients, renal function recovered spontaneously with conservative treatment. Histological examination of the kidney in 17 cases revealed acute tubular necrosis in 9, glomerulopathies in 4, and interstitial nephritis in 3, with 1 failing to show any pathologic alteration *(24)*.

Typical laboratory abnormalities of cholestatic hepatitis A include marked elevations of the serum bilirubin (often >10 mg/dl) and alkaline phosphatase (more than 2–3 times the upper limit of normal). In addition, the serum cholesterol may be elevated along with a minimal elevation of the AST and ALT. In most patients, the transaminases either decline abruptly or remain stable following the initial rise at the onset of the illness, whereas the serum bilirubin and alkaline phosphatase increase *(12,28)*. Peak bilirubin levels are reached at or following the eighth week of the illness. Jaundice and pruritus may last for 12 wk or more. IgM anti-HAV antibodies persist during the period of prolonged cholestasis. This condition usually resolves spontaneously and is followed by complete recovery. One study reported nine patients hospitalized with acute cholestatic viral hepatitis A. Jaundice lasted an average of 77 days (range: 30–120) and the total serum bilirubin concentration was a mean of 15.6 ± 10.8 mg/dl (range: 3–32.9 mg/dl). IgM anti-HAV was present in the serum for 6.3 ± 5.5 mo (median: 4, range: 2–19). Histopathological examination of the liver was performed in six patients. Most showed intralobular cholestasis and portal tract inflammation associated with dystrophy and paucity of bile ducts *(29)*.

Marked centrilobular cholestasis is the most common histologic finding in cholestatic hepatitis A *(12)*. In a series of 13 patients, 10 biopsies showed moderate to severe cholestasis consisting of bile thrombi, cholestatic liver cell rosettes, and ductular transformation of hepatocytes. In six cases, abnormal ductular epithelium was seen resembling the ductular lesion in septicemia, thought to be related to the accumulation of leukotrienes *(30)*.

Table 1
Characteristics of Viral and Alcoholic Cholestatic Hepatitis

Etiology	Risk factors	Clinical features	Laboratory abnormalities	Histology	Course	Treatment
Hepatitis A	None	Fever, anorexia, diarrhea, pruritus	IgM HAV, bilirubin> 10 g/dl, alkaline phosphatase> 2–3 times ULN, mild AST/ALT elevation	Centrilobular cholestasis, portal inflammation	Self-limiting. Rarely renal failure	Supportive. Steroids and UDCA questionable
Hepatitis B (FCH)	Immunosuppression including liver and other transplants	Rapidly progressive liver failure early after transplant, encephalopathy	Bilirubin> 10 g/dl, alkaline phosphatase> 2–3 times ULN, elevated INR, variable AST/ALT elevation, positive hepatitis B serology	Perisinusoidal fibrosis, cholestasis, ground-glass transformation, hepatocyte ballooning, mild mixed inflammatory reaction	Rapidly progressive with graft failure in weeks without treatment	Lamivudine, adefovir, ?entecavir
Hepatitis C (FCH)	Immunosuppression including liver and other transplants	Rapidly progressive liver failure early after	Bilirubin> 10 g/dl, alkaline phosphatase>	Perisinusoidal fibrosis, cholestasis, ground-glass	Rapidly progressive with graft failure in	? IFN and ribavirin but are usually not

		transplant, encephalopathy	2–3 times ULN, elevated INR, variable AST/ALT elevation, positive hepatitis C serology	transformation, hepatocyte ballooning, mild mixed inflammatory reaction	weeks. Retransplantation not successful	successful
Hepatitis C (VBDS)	Immunosuppression including liver and other transplants	Chronic cholestasis with progressive pruritus and ultimately liver failure 1–3 yr after transplant	Bilirubin> 10 g/dl, alkaline phosphatase> 2–3 times ULN, variable INR, elevated AST/ALT elevation, positive hepatitis C serology, negative AMA	Bile duct remnants and small bile duct loss	Variable but typically slowly progressive with graft failure	Reduction of immunosuppression may be attempted
Hepatitis E	None	Chronic jaundice, pruritus, nausea, lethargy	Bilirubin> 10 g/dl, alkaline phosphatase> 2–3 times ULN, mild AST/ALT	Bile plugs in the canaliculi, feathery degeneration of hepatocytes, liver cell rosettes,	Self-limiting. May last up to 6 mo. Rarely liver failure in pregnant females	Supportive

(Continued)

Table 1 (*Continued*)

Etiology	Risk factors	Clinical features	Laboratory abnormalities	Histology	Course	Treatment
			elevation, positive hepatitis E serology	lobular inflammation, and fatty changes of the hepatocytes		
CMV (FCH)	Immunosuppression including liver and other transplants	Rapidly progressive liver failure early after transplant, encephalopathy	Bilirubin> 10 g/dl, alkaline phosphatase> 2–3 times ULN, elevated INR, variable AST/ALT elevation, positive CMV serology	Perisinusoidal fibrosis, cholestasis, ground-glass transformation, hepatocyte ballooning, mild mixed inflammatory reaction	Rapidly progressive with graft failure in weeks	Reduction of immunosuppression, ? ganciclovir
EBV	None	Fever, jaundice, splenomegaly in young	Bilirubin> 10 g/dl, alkaline phosphatase> 2–3 times ULN, mild AST/ALT	Lymphocytic infiltration, granulomas and centrilobular cholestasis with minimal hepatocyte	Self-limiting. One case of liver failure reported	Supportive

			elevation, positive EBV serology	involvement		
Alcohol	None	Fever, anorexia, diarrhea, pruritus	Bilirubin> 10 g/dl, alkaline phosphatase> 2–3 times ULN, mild AST/ALT elevation	Focal bile stasis, neutrophilic infiltration of the perivenular areas, hepatocyte necrosis, ballooning and Mallory bodies, and pericellular fibrosis.	Cholestasis and degree of bilirubin elevation are indicators of poor prognosis	Steroids if discriminant function is more than 32

FCH, fibrosing cholestatic hepatitis; VBDS, vanishing bile duct syndrome.

A short course of corticosteroids may accelerate the resolution of pruritus and malaise and lead to lower serum bilirubin levels *(31)*. However, this approach was of no apparent benefit in one series *(12)* and may predispose to the development of the relapsing form of hepatitis A *(8)*. The benefits should be strongly weighed against the risk when considering treatment with corticosteroids *(32)*. The effect of ursodeoxycholic acid (UDCA) on acute viral hepatitis-related cholestasis has been studied . The study population consisted of 79 patients with acute viral hepatitis (HBV: 43, HCV: 11, HAV: 15, HEV: 3, Non A–E: 7) randomized to UDCA for 3 wk or no treatment. No significant difference in mean percentage decreases in transaminases between treated and untreated patients was found. By contrast, cholestatic indexes decreased significantly more in patients treated with UDCA than in controls. This effect was more evident in patients with increasing alanine transaminase levels at admission *(33)*. In light of this study, UDCA may be used for biochemical improvement; however, there is no effect on the course of the illness.

2.2. Hepatitis B

Fibrosing cholestatic hepatitis (FCH) is a severe form of hepatitis B (HBV) infection, usually seen in immunocompromised patients, such as liver allograft infection after liver transplantation for HBV or as a severe HBV reactivation induced by immunosuppression in patients with previously latent infection. In addition to liver transplant recipients, FCH has been reported in renal, heart, and bone marrow transplant recipients, AIDS patients, and other immunosuppressed patients with chronic HBV *(34–39)*.

Patients with FCH develop rapidly progressive liver failure. Without antiviral therapy, the condition is universally fatal within weeks of onset *(40)*. In an initial description, FCH was characterized histologically by thin, perisinusoidal bands of fibrosis extending from portal tracts to surrounding plates of ductular-type epithelium, prominent cholestasis, ground-glass transformation, and ballooning of hepatocytes with cell loss and a mild mixed inflammatory reaction. This was associated with prolongation of the prothrombin time, development of encephalopathy, and rapid graft failure in all patients, the earliest being at 2.5 mo, with all allografts lost in 9.5 mo *(41)*. FCH may be associated with a markedly increased rate of viral replication, with intracellular overexpression and massive accumulation of HBV antigens, resulting in direct cytopathic damage *(42–44)*.

Antiviral therapy with lamivudine or adefovir is standard treatment for FCH. Retransplantation may be necessary; however, recurrent FCH in subsequent allografts has been described (37,41,45). FCH has been treated successfully with lamivudine but the high probability of resistant mutants is a concern (46,47). However, since a direct cytopathic effect from rapid viral replication is the hallmark of FCH and escape mutants are usually replication deficient, FCH is rare in these patients. There are reports of FCH in patients with lamivudine-resistant HBV mutants. In such cases, a favorable outcome has been reported with the addition of adefovir, followed by retransplantation with adefovir and hepatitis B immunoglobulin prophylaxis (48–51).

2.3. Hepatitis C

Hepatitis C is associated with FCH following liver transplantation for hepatitis C and follows an aggressive course, similar to hepatitis B. This entity is characterized by early jaundice, cholestasis, and rapidly progressive fibrosis, leading to allograft loss within 3–6 mo of the transplant. Similar to hepatitis B-related FCH, FCH in hepatitis C also involves a direct cytopathic effect. Attempts at treatment with antiviral therapy and retransplantation lead to poor outcomes and usually fail (52–54). A case series of seven patients recommended indefinite treatment with IFN and ribavirin; however, additional studies with larger populations are needed before definitive recommendations can be made (55).

Hepatitis C has also been associated with the vanishing bile duct syndrome (VBDS), typically seen with chronic rejection of a liver allograft. In some cases, however, VBDS has been reported to be secondary to increased hepatitis C replication in the absence of rejection and a sudden increase in HCV-RNA levels. Histologically, the syndrome is characterized by cytoplasmic vacuolar degeneration and epithelial nuclear irregularity in small interlobular bile ducts in early stages and by bile duct remnants and bile duct loss in late stages. It has been shown to develop 1–3 yr following the transplant. The clinical course is variable and may be associated with a high mortality. VBDS is not limited to liver allograft recipients. In one study of renal transplant patients with hepatitis C, progressive VBDS developed in two of four patients, resulting in liver failure. The other two showed marked improvement after withdrawal of immunosuppression (56).

2.4. Hepatitis E

Hepatitis E virus (HEV) is an enteric virus usually associated with a self-resolving hepatitis. However, it may be fatal, especially in pregnant women. This disease is uncommon in the United States, except in the immigrant population. In rare instances, hepatitis E has been associated with cholestasis. Patients present with prolonged jaundice, pruritus, nausea, and lethargy. Laboratory abnormalities include marked elevations of the bilirubin and alkaline phosphatase, with milder elevations of the AST and ALT. A typical liver biopsy shows cholestasis with bile plugs in the canaliculi, feathery degeneration of hepatocytes and liver cell rosettes. In addition, lobular inflammation and fatty changes of the hepatocytes may be seen. Hepatitis E is usually self-limiting and may last 6 mo; however, it has been associated with liver failure in some reports *(57)*. Specifically, fulminant hepatic failure and cholestasis has been described with fatal outcome in pregnant women infected with hepatitis E *(58)*.

In a study of 24 hepatitis E patients, hepatitis E was more commonly associated with protracted cholestasis as compared to hepatitis A *(59)*. At day 7, 92% of hepatitis E patients had hyperbilirubinemia (median level of bilirubin 11.2 g/dl, range 1.6–66.5 g/dl) as compared to 72% of hepatitis A patients (median level of bilirubin 5.3 g/dl, range 0.6–52.8). At 4 wk, 58% of hepatitis E patients continued to have hyperbilirubinemia (median level of bilirubin 5.3 g/dl, range 1.3–41.7 g/dl) as compared to 32% of hepatitis A patients (median level of bilirubin 2.4 g/dl, range 0.9–56.8 g/dl). However, the study based cholestasis on levels of bilirubin, with no mention of the alkaline phosphatase levels. Supportive treatment is recommended.

2.5. Cytomegalovirus

FCH because of CMV is more common in immunosuppressed patients with clinical and histological characteristics similar to those described above. A decrease in immunosuppressive treatment usually leads to improvement. Treatment with ganciclovir has also been advocated, but is associated with a variable response *(35,60–62)*. A renal transplant recipient with cholestasis and the rapid development of liver failure and fatal outcome has been described. FCH was present histologically and acute CMV serologies were positive *(61)*.

2.6. Epstein–Barr Virus

Hepatic involvement with EBV is usually associated with mild transaminase elevations; however, it may also present as an acute cholestatic hepatitis *(63)*. Most patients present in their teens to twenties with fever, jaundice, and splenomegaly. Laboratory abnormalities include mild elevations of the AST and ALT. Total bilirubin is usually elevated significantly, at times more than 10 mg/dl, along with significant elevations of the alkaline phosphatase. Patients have positive serology for acute EBV infection. Liver biopsy is not required to establish the diagnosis; however, lymphocytic infiltration, granuloma formation, and centrilobular cholestasis with minimal hepatocyte involvement are seen *(64)*. The disease follows a self-limited course with spontaneous recovery in weeks and no treatment is indicated; however, one death has been reported from accelerated liver failure *(65–79)*.

3. CHOLESTATIC VARIANT OF ALCOHOLIC LIVER DISEASE

The association of alcoholic liver disease and cholestasis was first described by Mallory in 1911. He identified focal bile stasis as one of the features of alcoholic liver injury *(80)*. Subsequent studies showed the association of histologic cholestasis and jaundice with a poor prognosis *(81,82)*. Later studies established specific parameters with a poor prognosis in alcoholic liver disease. Malnutrition, an increased BUN and creatinine, the presence of encephalopathy, hyperbilirubinemia, and a prolonged prothrombin time are all markers of a poor outcome. Of these, a marked elevation of serum bilirubin levels, along with a prolonged prothrombin time, has been consistently shown to identify a subgroup of patients with a poor prognosis *(83–85)*. Maddrey's discriminant function (DF) identified patients with severe disease based on the prothrombin time and bilirubin *(83)*. The DF in its current modified form is calculated by: DF=4.6×[prothrombin time (s)–control prothrombin time (s)]+total bilirubin level (mg/dl) *(84)*. Patients with a DF greater than 32 have a 1-mo mortality level of 35–45% whereas those with a DF<32 have a 1-mo mortality level of 0–10% *(84,86,87)*. Although hyperbilirubinemia is frequently observed in alcoholic liver disease, histologic cholestasis is an uncommon finding. In a study of 36 patients with biopsy-proven alcoholic hepatitis, histological cholestasis was only present in 14 (38%) *(88)*. Another study of 306 chronic male alcoholics revealed 67 patients (22%) with moderate to severe cholestasis. In this study, the presence of histologic cholestasis was associated with a poor prognosis. Patients with alcoholic hepatitis and mild to absent cholestasis on liver biopsy had a 54% survival rate at 60 mo, whereas only 22% of patients with moderate to severe cholestasis survived *(89)*.

4. SUMMARY

Cholestatic variants of viral and alcoholic hepatitis are commonplace. Recognition of these variants may be crucial to the timely diagnosis and therapy of these disease states.

REFERENCES

1. Burgart LJ. Cholangitis in viral disease. Mayo Clin Proc 1998; 73: 479–482.
2. Eppinger H. (1937) *Die Leberkrankheiten: allgemeine und spezialle Pathologie und Therapie der Leber.* Julius Springer, Vienna.
3. Watson CJ and Hoffbauer W. The problem of prolonged hepatitis with particular reference to cholangiolitic cirrhosis of the liver. Ann Intern Med 1946; 25: 227.
4. Gall EA and Braunstein H. Hepatitis with manifestations simulating bile duct obstruction (so-called "cholangiolitic hepatitis"). Am J Clin Pathol 1955; 25: 1113–1127.
5. Ellakim M and Rachmilewitz M. Cholangiolitic manifestations in viral hepatitis. Gastroenterology 1956; 31: 369–383.
6. Sheldon S and Sherlock S. Viral hepatitis with features of prolonged bile retention. Br Med J 1957; 2: 734–738.
7. Dubin IN, Sullivan BH, LeGolvan PC, and Murphy LC. The cholestatic form of viral hepatitis. Am J Med 1960; 29: 55–72.
8. Schiff ER. A typical clinical manifestations of hepatitis A. Vaccine 1992; 10: S18–S20.
9. Verucchi G, Calza L, and Chiodo F. Viral hepatitis A with atypical course. Clinical, biochemical, and virologic study of 7 cases. Ann Ital Med Int 1999; 14: 239–245.
10. Ciocca M. Clinical course and consequences of hepatitis A infection. Vaccine 2000; 18: S71–S74.
11. Texeira MR, Jr, Weller IV, Murray M, et al. The pathology of hepatitis A in man. Liver 1982; 2: 53–60.
12. Gordon SC, Reddy KR, Schiff L, and Schiff ER. Prolonged intrahepatic cholestasis secondary to acute hepatitis A. Ann Intern Med 1984; 101: 635–637.
13. Kassas AL, Telegdy L, Mehesfalvi E, Szilagyi T, and Mihaly I. Polyphasic and protracted patterns of hepatitis A infection: a retrospective study. Acta Med Hung 1994; 50: 93–98.
14. Cvjetkovic D, Hrnjakovic Cvjetkovic I. Peripheral blood count disorders at the beginning of icteric phase of hepatitis A in adults according to clinical form. Miner Gastroenterol Dietol 2003; 49: 225–228.
15. Ibarra H, Riedemann S, Froesner G, et al. Natural history of viral hepatitis A in Chilean adults: clinical and laboratory aspects. GEN 1993; 47: 25–31.
16. Schiraldi O, Modugno A, Miglietta A, et al. Prolonged viral hepatitis type A with cholestasis: case report. Ital J Gastroenterol 1991; 23: 364.
17. Tong MJ el-Farra NS, and Grew MI. Clinical manifestations of hepatitis A: Recent experience in a community teaching hospital. J Infect Dis 1995; 171: S15–S18.

18. Agarwal KS, Puliyel JM, Mathew A, Lahoti D, and Gupta R. Acute pancreatitis with cholestatic hepatitis: an unusual manifestation of hepatitis A. Ann Trop Paediatr 1999; 19: 391–394.

19. Ilan Y, Hillman M, Oren R, Zlotogorski A, and Shouval D. Vasculitis and cryoglobulinemia associated with persisting cholestatic hepatitis A virus infection. Am J Gastroenterol 1990; 85: 586–587.

20. Werblowsky-Constantini N, Livshin R, Burstein M, Zeligowski A, and Tur-Kaspa R. Toxic epidermal necrolysis associated with acute cholestatic viral hepatitis A. J Clin Gastroenterol 1989; 11: 691–693.

21. Jamil SM and Massry SG. Acute anuric renal failure in nonfulminant hepatitis A infection. Am J Nephrol 1998; 18: 329–332.

22. Malbrain MLNG, DeMeester X, Wilmer AP, et al. Another case of acute renal failure due to acute tubular necrosis (ATN), proven by renal biopsy in nonfulminant hepatitis A (HAV) infection. Nephrol Dial Transplant 1997; 12: 1543–1544.

23. Faust RL and Pimstone N. Acute renal failure associated with nonfulminant hepatitis A viral infection. Am J Gastroenterol 1996; 91: 369–372.

24. McCann UG, II, Rabito F, Shah M, Nolan CR, III, and Lee M. Acute renal failure complicating nonfulminant hepatitis A. West J Med 1996; 165: 308–310.

25. Lin CC, Chang CH, Lee SH, Chiang SS, and Yang AA. Acute renal failure in non-fulminant hepatitis A. Nephrol Dial Transplant 1996; 11: 2061–2066.

26. Odutola TA and Amira O. Non-oliguric acute renal failure in non-fulminant acute viral hepatitis. Nephrol Dial Transplant 1998; 13: 814–815.

27. Wolf M, Oneta CM, Jornod P, et al. Cholestatic hepatitis A complicated by acute renal insufficiency. Z Gastroenterol 2001; 39: 519–522.

28. Duncan CR, Palmitano JB, Tani RD, and Viola LA. Cholestatic viral hepatitis: is it an easy diagnosis? Acta Gastroenterol Latinoam 1985; 15: 225–231.

29. Corpechot C, Cadranel JF, Hoang C, et al. Cholestatic viral hepatitis A in adults. Clinical, biological and histopathological study of 9 cases. Gastroenterol Clin Biol 1994; 18: 743–750.

30. Sciot R, Van Damme B, and Desmet VJ. Cholestatic features in hepatitis A. J Hepatol 1986; 3: 172–181.

31. Terrault NA and Wright TL. Viral hepatitis A through G. In: Gastrointestinal and Liver Disease (Feldman M, Scharschmidt BF, and Sleisenger MH, Eds), WB Saunders, Philadelphia, 1998; p. 1129.

32. Cuthbert JA. Hepatitis A: old and new. Clin Microbiol Rev 2001; 14: 38–58.

33. Fabris P, Tositti G, Mazzella G, et al. Effect of ursodeoxycholic acid administration in patients with acute viral hepatitis: a pilot study. Aliment Pharmacol Ther 1999; 13: 1187–1193.

34. Chen CH, Chen PJ, Chu JS, Yeh KH, Lai MY, and Chen DS. Fibrosing cholestatic hepatitis in a hepatitis B surface antigen carrier after renal transplantation. Gastroenterology 1994; 107: 1514–1518.

35. Duseja A, Nada R, Kalra N, et al. Fibrosing cholestatic hepatitis-like syndrome in a hepatitis B virus and hepatitis C virus-negative renal transplant recipient: a case report with autopsy findings. Trop Gastroenterol. 2003; 24: 31–34.

36. Poulet B, Chapel F, Deny P, et al. Fibrosing cholestatic hepatitis by B virus reactivation in AIDS. Ann Pathol 1996; 16: 188–191.

37. Fang JW, Wright TL, and Lau JY. Fibrosing cholestatic hepatitis in patient with HIV and hepatitis B. Lancet 1993; 342: 1175.

38. Cooksley WG and McIvor CA. Fibrosing cholestatic hepatitis and HBV after bone marrow transplantation. Biomed Pharmacother 1995; 49: 117–124.

39. McIvor C, Morton J, Bryant A, Cooksley WG, Durrant S, and Walker N. Fatal reactivation of precore mutant hepatitis B virus associated with fibrosing cholestatic hepatitis after bone marrow transplantation. Ann Intern Med 1994; 121: 274–275.

40. O'Grady JG, Smith HM, Davies SE, et al. Hepatitis B virus reinfection after orthotopic liver transplantation. Serological and clinical implications. J Hepatol 1992; 14: 104–111.

41. Davies SE, Portmann BC, O'Grady JG, et al. Hepatic histological findings after transplantation for chronic hepatitis B virus infection, including a unique pattern of fibrosing cholestatic hepatitis. Hepatology 1991; 13: 150–157.

42. Benner KG, Lee RG, Keeffe EB, Lopez RR, Sasaki AW, and Pinson CW. Fibrosing cytolytic liver failure secondary to recurrent hepatitis B after liver transplantation. Gastroenterology 1992; 103: 1307–1312.

43. Mason AL, Wick M, White HM, et al. Increased hepatocyte expression of hepatitis B virus transcription in patients with features of fibrosing cholestatic hepatitis. Gastroenterology 1993; 105: 237–244.

44. Lau JY, Bain VG, Davies SE, et al. High-level expression of hepatitis B viral antigens in fibrosing cholestatic hepatitis. Gastroenterology 1992; 102: 956–962.

45. Brind AM, Bennett MK, and Bassendine MF. Nucleotide analogue therapy in fibrosing cholestatic hepatitis—a case report in an HBsAg positive renal transplant recipient. Liver 1998; 18: 134–139.

46. Chan T-M, Wu P-C, Li F-K, et al. Treatment of fibrosing cholestatic hepatitis with lamivudine. Gastroenterology 1998; 115: 177–181.

47. Faraidy KA, Yoshida EM, Davis GE, et al. Alteration of the dismal natural history of fibrosing cholestatic hepatitis secondary to hepatitis B virus with the use of lamivudine. Transplantation 1997; 64: 926–928.

48. Lo CM, Cheung ST, Ng IO, Liu CL, Lai CL, and Fan ST. Fibrosing cholestatic hepatitis secondary to precore/core promoter hepatitis B variant with lamivudine resistance: successful retransplantation with combination adefovir dipivoxil and hepatitis B immunoglobulin. Liver Transplant 2004; 10: 557–563.

49. Walsh KM, Woodall T, Lamy P, Wight DG, Bloor S, and Alexander GJ. Successful treatment with adefovir dipivoxil in a patient with fibrosing cholestatic hepatitis and lamivudine resistant hepatitis B virus. Gut 2001; 49: 436–440.

50. Beckebaum S, Malago M, Dirsch O, et al. Efficacy of combined lamivudine and adefovir dipivoxil treatment for severe HBV graft reinfection after living donor liver transplantation. Clin Transplant 2003; 17: 554–559.

51. Tillmann HL, Bock CT, Bleck JS, et al. Successful treatment of fibrosing cholestatic hepatitis using adefovir dipivoxil in a patient with cirrhosis and renal insufficiency. Liver Transplant 2003; 9: 191–196.

52. Schugler L, Sheiner P, Thung S, et al. Severe recurrent hepatitis C following orthotopic liver transplantation. Hepatology 1996; 23: 971–976.

53. Dickson RC, Caldwell SH, Ishitani MB, Lau JYN, Driscoll CJ, and Stevenson WC. Clinical and histologic patterns in early graft failure due to recurrent hepatitis C infection after liver transplantation. Transplantation 1996; 61: 701–705.

54. Doughty AL, Spencer JD, Cossart YE, and McCaughan GW. Cholestatic hepatitis post liver transplant is associated with persistingly high serum hepatitis C viral loads. Liver Transplant Surg 1998; 4: 15–21.

55. Gopal DV and Rosen HR. Duration of antiviral therapy for cholestatic HCV recurrence may need to be indefinite. Liver Transplant 2003; 9: 348–353.

56. Boletis JN, Delladetsima JK, Makris F, et al. Cholestatic syndromes in renal transplant recipients with HCV infection. Transplant Int 2000; 13: S375–S379.

57. Mechnik L, Bergman N, Attali M, et al. Acute hepatitis E virus infection presenting as a prolonged cholestatic jaundice. J Clin Gastroenterol 2001; 33: 421–422.
58. Asher LV, Innis BL, Shrestha MP, Ticehurst J, and Baze WB. Virus-like particles in the liver of a patient with fulminant hepatitis and antibody to hepatitis E virus. J Med Viro 1990; 31: 229–233.
59. Chau TN, Lai ST, Tse C, et al. Epidemiology and Clinical Features of Sporadic Hepatitis E as Compared with Hepatitis A. Am J Gastroenterol 2006; 101: 292–296.
60. Serna-Higuera C, Gonzalez-Garcia M, Milicua JM, and Munoz V. Acute cholestatic hepatitis by cytomegalovirus in an immunocompetent patient resolved with ganciclovir. J Clin Gastroenterol 1999; 29: 276–277.
61. Agarwal SK, Kalra V, Dinda A, et al. Fibrosing cholestatic hepatitis in renal transplant recipient with CMV infection: a case report. Int Urol Nephrol 2004; 36: 433–435.
62. Munoz de Bustillo E, Benito A, Colina F, et al. Fibrosing cholestatic hepatitis-like syndrome in hepatitis B virus—negative and hepatitis C virus—negative renal transplant recipients. Am J Kidney Dis 2001; 38: 640–645.
63. Horwitz CA, Burke MD, Grimes P, et al. Hepatic function in mononucleosis induced by Epstein–Barr virus and cytomegalovirus. Clin Chem 1980; 26: 243–246.
64. Mandell GL, Bennett JE, and Dolin R. Epstein–Barr virus, Princ Prac. Infect Dis 2000; 2: 1601–1602.
65. Dinulos J, Mitchell DK, Egerton J, et al. Hydrops of the gallbladder associated with Epstein–Barr virus infection: a report of two cases and review of the literature. Pediatr. Infect Dis J 1994; 13: 924–929.
66. Edoute Y, Baruch Y, Lachte J, et al. Severe cholestatic jaundice induced by Epstein–Barr virus infection in the elderly. J Gastroenterol Hepatol 1998; 13: 821–824.
67. Bernstein CN and Minuk GY. Infectious mononucleosis presenting with cholestatic liver disease. Ann Intern Med 1998; 128: 509.
68. Hinedi TB and Koff RS. Cholestatic hepatitis induced by Epstein–Barr virus infection in an adult. Dig Dis Sci 2003; 48: 539–541.
69. Yuge A, Kinoshita E, Moriuchi M, et al. Persistent hepatitis associated with chronic active Epstein–Barr virus infection. Pediatr Infect Dis J 2004; 23: 74–76.
70. Barlow G, Kilding R, and Green ST. Epstein–Barr virus infection mimicking extra hepatic biliary obstruction. J R Soc Med 2003; 93: 316–318.
71. Sung RY, Peck R, and Murray HG. Persistent high fever and gall-bladder wall thickening in a child with primary Epstein–Barr viral infection, Aust Paediatr J 1989; 25: 368–369.
72. Valentini P, Angelone DF, Miceli Sopo S, et al. Cholestatic jaundice in infectious mononucleosis. Miner Pediatr 2000; 52: 303–306.
73. Cotton WK, McFadden JW, and Walls LL. Case report: atypical presentation of cholestatic jaundice. Postgrad Med 1976; 60: 259–261.
74. O'Donovan N and Fitzgerald E. Gallbladder wall thickening in infectious mononucleosis: an ominous sign. Postgrad Med J 1996; 72: 299–300.
75. Ghosh A, Ghoshal UC, Kochhar R, et al. Infectious mononucleosis hepatitis: report of two patients. Indian J Gastroenterol 1997; 16: 113–114.
76. Kimura H, Nagasaka T, Hoshino Y, et al. Severe hepatitis caused by Epstein–Barr virus without infection of hepatocytes. Hum Pathol 2001; 32: 757–762.
77. Deutsch M, Dourakis SP, Sevastianos VA, et al. Deep jaundice in an adolescent, Postgrad Med J 2003; 79: 548–549.

78. Massei F, Palla G, Ughi C, et al. Cholestasis as a presenting feature of acute Epstein–Barr virus infection. Pediatr Infect Dis J 2001; 20: 721–722.
79. Tahan V, Ozaras R, Uzunismail H, et al. Infectious mononucleosis presenting with severe cholestatic liver disease in the elderly. J Clin Gastroenterol 2001; 33: 88–89.
80. Mallory F. Cirrhosis of the liver. Five different types of lesions from which it may arise. Bull Johns Hopkins Hosp 1911; 22: 69–75.
81. Phillips GB and Davidson CS. Acute hepatic insufficiency of the chronic alcoholic. Clinical and pathologic study. Arch Intern Med 1954; 94: 585–603.
82. Beckett AG, Livingstone AV, and Hill KR. Acute alcoholic hepatitis. Br Med J 1961; 2: 1113–1119.
83. Maddrey WC, Boitnott JK, Bedine MS, Weber FL, Mezey E, and White RI. Corticosteroid therapy of alcoholic hepatitis. Gastroenterology 1978; 75: 193–199.
84. Carithers RL, Jr, Herlong HF, Diehl AM, et al. Methylprednisolone therapy in patients with severe alcoholic hepatitis: a randomized multicenter trial. Ann Intern Med 1989; 110: 685–690.
85. Maddrey WC. Is therapy with testosterone or anabolic-androgenic steroids useful in the treatment of alcoholic liver disease? Hepatology 1986; 6: 1033–1035.
86. Ramond MJ, Poynard T, Rueff B, et al. A randomized trial of prednisolone in patients with severe alcoholic hepatitis. N Engl J Med 1992; 326: 507–512.
87. Mathurin P, Mendenhall CL, Carithers RL, et al. Corticosteroids improve short-term survival in patients with severe alcoholic hepatitis (AH): individual data analysis of the last three randomized placebo controlled double blind trials of corticosteroids in severe AH. J Hepatol 2002; 36: 480–487.
88. Trinchet JC, Gerhardt MF, Balkau B, Munz C, and Poupon RE. Serum bile acids and cholestasis in alcoholic hepatitis. Relationship with usual liver tests and histological features. J Hepatol 1994; 21: 235–240.
89. Nissenbaum M, Chedid A, and Mendenhal C. For the VA Cooperative Study Group #119. Prognostic significance of cholestatic alcoholic hepatitis. Dig Dis Sci. 1990; 35: 891–896.

8   Cholestatic Liver Disease Related to Systemic Disorders

Kimberly Forde and David E. Kaplan

CONTENTS

Abstract

Cholestasis frequently results from systemic disorders in which the hepatic involvement is secondary or indirect. The objective of this chapter is to review major systemic conditions that are associated with cholestasis in terms of epidemiology, pathophysiology, presentations, and possible treatment. Conditions will be discussed in terms of the likely anatomic level of involvement e.g. at the level of the canaliculus, the intralobular ductules, and large intrahepatic bile ducts, emphasizing and highlighting common aspects of the pathophysiology of several of these processes.

Key Words: Cholestasis of sepsis; intrahepatic cholestasis of pregnancy; sarcoidosis; cystic fibrosis; Stauffer's syndrome.

1. INTRODUCTION

As detailed in the preceding chapters, predominantly hepatic processes such as infection by hepatotrophic viruses, poisoning by hepatotoxins, autoimmune liver disease, and biliary genetic disorders

From: *Clinical Gastroenterology: Cholestatic Liver Disease*
Edited by: K. D. Lindor and J. A. Talwalkar © Humana Press Inc., Totowa, NJ

result in cholestasis as part of the primary pathophysiology. By contrast, in many systemic disorders hepatic involvement is secondary or indirect yet manifests with varying degrees of cholestasis. The aim of this chapter is to review the epidemiology, pathophysiology, manifestations, and appropriate therapies of the major systemic conditions that are associated with cholestasis.

Conditions to be discussed will include processes that disrupt the concentration of bile contents within biliary canaliculi such as sepsis, hyperestrogenic states, and congestive heart failure; processes that predominantly disrupt bile flow within intralobular ductules such as sarcoidosis, cystic fibrosis (CF), and portal metastastic disease; and finally processes that disrupt bile flow in large intrahepatic bile ducts. Paraneoplastic cholestasis (Stauffer's syndrome), a rare cause of cholestasis associated with extrahepatic malignancy, will also be discussed.

2. CHOLESTASIS RESULTING FROM IMPAIRED CANALICULAR FUNCTION

Bile formation is a highly ordered process incorporating the active movement of solutes across a polarized membrane in hepatocytes *(1)*. This is characterized by the stepwise movement of bile salts, inorganic, and organic solutes via transmembrane protein transporters across the canalicular surface *(1,2)*. Canalicular cholestasis results from disruption of the number and/or function of hepatocyte protein transporters. Certain systemic aberrancies such as sepsis, hyperestrogenemia, and congestive heart failure disrupt bile synthesis causing clinical cholestatic syndromes.

2.1. Cholestasis of Sepsis

Despite the lack of direct liver involvement, extrahepatic bacterial infections may indirectly result in liver dysfunction. This condition, designated the cholestasis of sepsis, often manifests with jaundice and associated elevations in serum bilirubin, alkaline phosphatase, and γ-glutamyl transpeptidase levels *(3,4)*. Mild cholestasis may occur very early in the course of systemic infections, preceding bacteriologic diagnosis in up to a third of patients *(4)*. Experimental models demonstrate the impairment of bile acid transport from the effects of bacterial lipopolysaccharide (LPS) endotoxins. Released into the portal or systemic circulation, LPS directly stimulates hepatic macrophages to produce inflammatory mediators such as tumor necrosis factor, interleukin-1, interleukin-6, and nitric oxide *(5)*. These mediators alter the expression of various bile transport proteins within hepatocyte *(5–9)*.

The diagnosis of cholestasis of sepsis is generally made clinically after exclusion of extrahepatic obstruction. Liver biopsy, if obtained, reveals bland cholestasis ("cholestasis lenta") characterized by dilated cholangioles with bile plugs without associated inflammation or hepatocyte injury *(10)*. Other nonspecific pathologic findings include mild portal mononuclear infiltrate, fatty changes, or Kupffer cell hyperplasia *(11,12)*. Treatment is supportive, including management of the underlying septic state with directed antimicrobial therapy and hemodynamic stabilization. In experimental models, dexamethasone attenuates the effect of LPS on mRNA levels of transporters, subcellular distribution of transporters, and solute excretion *(9)* suggesting a theoretical role for corticosteroid therapy in cholestasis of sepsis.

2.2. Estrogen-Mediated Cholestasis

An association between oral contraceptive (OCP) use and cholestasis was first appreciated in the 1960s *(13–15)* with subsequent recognition of intrahepatic cholestasis of pregnancy (ICP) *(15)*. Studies in small animal and in vitro models have confirmed that estrogens inhibit the bile acid-independent component of bile flow as well as by altering bile salt excretion *(15)*. Estrogen also directly inhibits bile salt transport by canalicular vesicles via interactions with proteins such as the bile salt export pump (BSEP) and Mrp2 *(16–18)*.

ICP, the most common hepatic disease associated with pregnancy, is a usually benign disorder associated with pruritus and cholestatic liver enzyme abnormalities during the second and third trimester of pregnancy. These manifestations resolve within 2–3 wk postpartum. Ten percent of patients develop jaundice *(19)*. Whereas liver biopsy is rarely required for diagnosis, the characteristic histological feature of ICP is cholestasis with bile plugs localized to zone 3 *(20)*.

ICP tends to cluster in kindreds and in particular regions such as Chile, Bolivia, and Sweden *(15)* suggesting a genetic predisposition to the effects of estrogen on biliary transport. Investigation into the role of mutations in biliary transport-related genes has shown that up to 15% of cases are associated with heterozygosity for mutations in the ABCB4/MDR3 bile acid transporter gene *(21–25)*. Mutations in other bile acid transporters such as FIC1 *(22,26,27)* and BSEP *(22)* have also been implicated. As a consequence of its relationship to hormone levels and genetics, ICP recurs in 60–70% of subsequent pregnancies *(19)*.

Whereas maternal peripartum morbidity and mortality are not significantly altered, ICP is associated with an increased rate of fetal prematurity and death *(28)*. Despite the resolution of cholestasis after delivery, patients remain at increased lifetime risk of gallstones and gallstone-related complications *(29)*.

Treatment with ursodeoxycholic acid (UDCA) has been shown to reduce pruritus, improve liver-associated enzymes, *(28,30–39)*, and to improve fetal outcomes *(31,38)*. Agents such as S-adenosylmethionine *(33)* and cholestyramine *(31)*, either alone or in combination with UDCA, have proven less effective than UDCA. Therefore, UDCA is widely considered the primary treatment modality for ICP.

2.3. Cholestasis Resulting from Hepatic Congestion

Whereas cardiogenic shock is associated with ischemic liver injury characterized by markedly elevated, rapidly normalizing aminotransferase levels during the recovery phase, chronic heart failure is frequently associated with predominantly cholestatic liver enzyme abnormalities *(40–44)*. These abnormalities are often associated with more severe heart failure *(45,46)* and increased cardiac mortality *(43,44)*. Laboratory studies typically reveal a mild-to-moderate elevation in total bilirubin, (predominantly unconjugated), mild alterations in serum aminotransferase levels, prominent elevation in γ-glutamyl transferase, and moderate increases in alkaline phosphatase *(43)*. There may also be modest prolongation of the prothrombin time. Prolonged passive congestion of the liver can lead to pericentral fibrosis with eventual central–central bridging fibrosis *(42)*, termed cardiac sclerosis.

The underlying mechanism by which heart failure causes cholestasis is poorly understood. Whereas it has been speculated that a relative sensitivity of the bile ducts to chronic hypoperfusion could be responsible *(40, 42,43)*, a study of congested hepatocytes under electron microscopy suggests that increases of intrasinusoidal pressure might disrupt the zonula occludens between neighboring hepatocytes. This creates a shunt between the canaliculus and the sinusoid allowing efflux of bile contents back into the systemic circulation *(40)*. These findings require confirmation, but provide a simple yet elegant explanation for this phenomenon.

2.4. Paraneoplastic Cholestasis (Stauffer's Syndrome)

Paraneoplastic cholestasis, first described by Stauffer in 1961 in a patient with renal cell carcinoma *(47)*, is characterized by elevations in alkaline phosphatase often with jaundice and pruritus in the absence of biliary obstruction or evident hepatic metastases *(48–52)*. An association with abnormal prothrombin times because of low-grade disseminated intravascular coagulation has been reported *(53)*. Histological series demonstrate a nonobstructive sinusoidal dilation of unclear significance in some patients with Stauffer's syndrome *(54)*. Typically, surgical resection or other treatment of the primary tumor leads to resolution of cholestasis *(48,49,51,55)*. The pathogenesis of paraneoplastic cholestasis remains unclear but inflammatory cytokines such as interleukin-6 *(56,57)* and interleukin-1β *(58)* have been implicated. In vitro, these cytokines alter expression of hepatocyte bile acid transporters *(59,60)* and therefore this condition most likely shares pathophysiological features with the cholestasis of sepsis. Therapeutic blockade of interleukin-6 led to attenuation of cholestasis in one series *(56)*, strengthening the pathological role of inflammatory cytokines in this disorder. Although most commonly associated with renal cell carcinoma *(48–50,56,61)*, Stauffer's syndrome has been reported with prostate adenocarcinoma *(55,62)*, pheochromocytoma *(58)*, medullary thyroid cancer *(63)*, and systemic mastocytosis *(64)*.

3. CHOLESTASIS RESULTING FROM OBSTRUCTION OF SMALL INTRAHEPATIC BILE DUCTS

As bile exits the canaliculus, it enters the larger terminal bile ductules and subsequently into a network of interlobular bile ducts *(65)*. These interlobular ducts run adjacent to portal vein branches and are therefore sensitive to systemic processes that cause inflammation in or invade portal tracts.

3.1. Sarcoidosis

Sarcoidosis, a multiorgan disorder characterized by the presence of noncaseating granulomas within various organs, primarily causes lung disease but may affect any solid organ. The disease affects persons of all ethnicities and ages but the highest incidence rates are noted in African-American women aged 30–39 yr *(66)*. The pathophysiology, while not well understood, is thought to involve an aberrant host immune response to an unknown, possibly environmental, antigen in a predisposed host *(67)*. Subsequently, macrophages and lymphocytes are activated under the influence of inflammatory cytokines, convert into epitheliod histiocytes, organize into clusters, and form noncaseating granulomas *(68)* which destroy the underlying parenchyma. Recent case reports of *de novo* sarcoidosis following treatment for chronic hepatitis C *(69,70)* suggest that interferon-alpha may also initiate sarcoidosis lesions in the liver.

The presence of sarcoid granulomas in the liver occurs in approximately 75% of cases of systemic sarcoidosis *(71–73)*. For unknown reasons, granulomas of sarcoidosis preferentially form within portal triads *(74,75)* but can also occur in the parenchyma *(76)*. Progressive accumulation of portal and periportal granulomas eventually results in destruction of the interlobular bile ducts which eventually leads to a chronic cholestatic syndrome in a minority of patients *(75,77)*. Less commonly, sarcoidosis involves *(78)*, larger intrahepatic ducts causing a primary sclerosing cholangitis (PSC)-like presentation *(79,80)*, or causes acute liver failure because of sarcoid vasculitis-induced Budd–Chiari syndrome *(81,82)*. In cholestatic patients, serum chemistries typically demonstrate an elevated alkaline phosphatase (2–30 fold), moderately elevated total bilirubin, and aminotransferase levels, increased cholesterol, and mild hyper-gammaglobulinemia *(78)*. Histology usually reveals noncaseating granulomas, bile plugs, and varying degrees of bile duct destruction *(74,78)*. Advanced cases will reveal severe ductopenia, cirrhosis, and in some cases dense periportal fibrosis similar to PSC *(74,78,83)*.

Early symptomatic hepatic sarcoidosis is clinically similar to primary biliary cirrhosis (PBC) with or without manifestations of noncirrhotic portal hypertension *(78,84–87)*. Although steroid therapy is the mainstay of treatment for pulmonary sarcoidosis, little data exist to validate or disprove their benefit in hepatic sarcoidosis. Whereas individual case series suggest that liver enzymes may improve *(88–90)*, others suggest that these improvements do not alter the natural history of the disease *(91,92)*. Other therapies reported to have anecdotal efficacy include UDCA *(93)*, chlorambucil *(94)*, and chloroquine *(95)*.

In advanced cases complicated by decompensated cirrhosis or refractory complications of portal hypertension, liver transplantation may be required *(96–99)*. Although uncommonly necessary, survival is excellent. In one single-center series, 0.3% of adult liver transplants were performed because of hepatic sarcoidosis with a 100% one-year and 86% five-year survival *(97)*. Whereas the immunosuppression required for liver transplantation would be expected to suppress granuloma formation, cases of recurrent sarcoid manifestations requiring corticosteroids have been described *(96,98)*.

3.2. Cystic Fibrosis

CF is an autosomal recessive disorder that affects 1 in 2000 Caucasian children. CF is characterized by mutations in the cystic fibrosis transmembrane conductance receptor (CFTR), a chloride channel critical for transport of electrolytes in various organs, including the liver and biliary tree. The pathogenesis of liver disease in CF is characterized by the accumulation of mucinous secretions within intrahepatic bile ducts lined by biliary epithelium, the primary cell type shown to express

CFTR *(100)*. It has been traditionally thought that focal obstruction incites inflammation which induces bile ductular proliferation and fibrosis *(101–104)*. The role of obstruction and inflammation in this process has recently been questioned *(100)*. Direct toxicity of bile salts to biliary epithelial cells has been proposed as an alternative explanation *(100)*.

Approximately 25–41% of CF patients develop clinically apparent hepatobiliary disease *(105–107)* with a peak prevalence at approximately age 12 *(107)*. Disease manifestations include neonatal cholestasis, fatty infiltration of the liver, and biliary obstruction from inspissated secretions. Eventual biliary cirrhosis with an incidence of approximately 4.5% per year of CF-related liver disease may develop *(105)*. CF patients with biochemical evidence of liver disease are generally treated with high-dose UDCA, a therapy that has been shown to improve liver enzymes and stabilize disease in studies reporting up to 10 yr of follow-up *(108–114)*. CF-related liver disease is an infrequent indication for liver transplantation. A study of 10 pediatric liver transplantation patients, which comprised 3.5% of the overall transplant population at a large US pediatric transplant center, demonstrated high mortality (40%) in the first 2 yr after transplantation because of pulmonary complications *(115)*. Given the special cardiopulmonary problems of the CF population, some experts strongly favor medical and endoscopic therapies for portal hypertension *(116,117)*.

3.3. Rheumatologic Disease

The incidence of cholestatic liver enzyme abnormalities in rheumatoid disorders is highly variable, with elevations of alkaline phosphatase noted in up to 62% of polymyalgia rheumatica patients *(118)*, 6 to 45% in rheumatoid arthritis (RA) *(119–123)*, and up to 42% Felty's syndrome *(124,125)*. The cause of cholestatic liver enzyme abnormalities in these conditions is poorly characterized, but nonspecific portal inflammation has been shown to occur frequently in RA *(126)*. Whereas symptomatic cholestasis is rare in most rheumatologic disorders, concomitant PBC develops in 1-15% of patients *(119,127)*. In this setting, UDCA effectively treats the PBC-related cholestasis but has no effect on the primary autoimmune disorder *(128)*.

Cholestasis may also result from therapies for rheumatologic conditions. For example, prolonged cholestasis with ductopenia has been observed following the use of gold salts for the treatment of RA *(129–131)*. Drug-induced cholestasis has also been implicated with D-penicillamine *(132,133)* and sulfasalazine therapy *(134)*.

3.4. Extrahepatic Malignancies
that Obstruct Small Intrahepatic Ducts

Whereas malignancies such as melanoma, breast, lung, and colon cancer often metastasize to the liver and establish focal lesions that disrupt bile flow, infiltrating malignancies such as Hodgkin's disease (HD) and non-Hodgkin's lymphoma (NHL) result in cholestatic disease by obstructing small interlobular ducts *(135,136)*. Liver involvement with these malignancies is common, occurring in 11–80% of HD patients undergoing diagnostic laparotomy *(137–139)* and in 24–40% of NHL cases *(138,140,141)*. HD in particular is associated with progressive inflammatory lesions within portal tracts, eventually resulting in ductopenia (also known as vanishing bile duct syndrome) *(142–148)*, Which is associated with a dismal prognosis *(142,143,148)*. Whereas HD rarely obstructs the extrahepatic biliary system by enlarged porta hepatis lymph nodes *(149)*, extrahepatic obstruction is the most commonly reported source of jaundice in NHL *(150)*. By contrast, chronic intrahepatic cholestasis related to NHL is not reported, possibly because of a more aggressive and fulminant course of hepatic NHL *(151–153)*.

3.5. GVHD

Graft versus host disease (GVHD), one of the primary complications of allogeneic hematopoietic stem cell transplantation, frequently involves the liver resulting in acute and chronic cholestatic disease. In animal models, GVHD appears to be mediated by influx of $CD8^+$ T cells into portal tracts resulting in nonsuppurative destructive cholangitis *(154)*. In human series, bile ductulitis evolves from 35 to 90 d posttransplant, after which point biopsies begin to show portal fibrosis and bile duct loss *(155)*. Significant acute GVHD, which occurs in 35–50% of allogeneic BMT patients *(156,157)*, involves the liver in approximately 25% of patients *[158]* with elevations in alkaline phosphatase and bilirubin. In approximately one-third of cases, there may also be associated marked increases in aminotransferase levels *(157,159)*. Acute hepatic GVHD usually resolves with immunosuppressive therapy, but progresses to chronic hepatic GVHD in a subset of patients *(160,161)*. Chronic GVHD, a chronic cholestatic syndrome, shares many clinical and pathological features with PBC *(162)*, raising interest in common pathophysiological mechanisms *(163,164)* and therapeutic agents *(165)*. Despite that 60–80% of BMT patients develop some degree of chronic GVHD *(156,161, 166,167)*, progressive liver fibrosis and evolution to cirrhosis is fairly uncommon. When cirrhosis occurs, it is usually because of coincident chronic viral infection *(168)*.

4. CHOLESTASIS RESULTING FROM OBSTRUCTION OF LARGE INTRAHEPATIC BILE DUCTS

Various systemic conditions lead primarily to structuring of large intrahepatic and extrahepatic bile ducts resembling PSC. AIDS cholangiopathy and floxuridine (FUDR)-induced biliary injury will be discussed briefly as examples.

4.1. AIDS Cholangiopathy

AIDS-related cholangiopathy, a consequence of underlying opportunistic infections of the biliary epithelium, presents with fever, right upper quadrant pain, and elevation in alkaline phosphatase associated with CMV and cryptosporidium infections *(169,170)*. Three-quarters of patients have abnormal cholangiograms with biliary lesions such as sclerosing cholangitis, papillary stenosis, and/or extrahepatic strictures *(171,172)*. Histologically, AIDS cholangiopathy is characterized by a periductal mixed inflammatory infiltrate and ductal dilatation *(170)*. Because of the advanced stage of AIDS at the time of development of this complication, the prognosis remains poor despite temporizing interventions such as endoscopic retrograde cholangiopancreatography (ERCP) and antimicrobial therapy *(173)*.

4.2. Iatrogenic Sclerosing Cholangiopathy

Starting in the mid-1980s, intrahepatic arterial infusion of chemotherapeutic agents such as floxuridine (FUDR) was employed for the treatment of focal colorectal liver metastases *(174–176)*. FUDR infusion resulted in an ischemic ductal injury, with the formation of strictures limited to the large intrahepatic ducts with a relative sparing of the common bile duct *(177)*. On cholangiography, FUDR-related injury resembled PSC with large duct involvement *(178–180)*. Biliary stenting after FUDR infusions can relieve some degree of obstruction but often cannot address all of the affected small biliary radicles *(176)* resulting in chronic cholestatic disease.

5. SUMMARY AND CONCLUSION

Many disorders profoundly alter biliary function and induce cholestatic syndromes. These effects range from disruption of function of the smallest bile canaliculi to obstruction of bile ducts of all sizes within the liver. In general, canalicular cholestasis results from inflammatory or hormonal mediators which cause alteration in bile acid transporter expression or function. Genetic variations in bile salt transport proteins may impact the expression of disease, and therapeutic reduction of the precipitating mediator, e.g., antimicrobial therapy, tumor debulking, partuition, leads to clinical resolution. By contrast, systemic diseases that affect small intralobular and larger intrahepatic bile ducts tend to resemble PBC and PSC clinically, histologically, and often radiologically. These conditions unfortunately tend to be destructive and progressive.

REFERENCES

1. Moseley RH. Sepsis and cholestasis. Clin Liver Dis 1999; 3(3): 465–475.
2. Trauner M, Meier PJ, and Boyer JL. Molecular pathogenesis of cholestasis. N Engl J Med 1998; 339(17): 1217–1227.
3. Tung CB, Tung CF, Yang DY, et al. Extremely high levels of alkaline phosphatase in adult patients as a manifestation of bacteremia. Hepatogastroenterology 2005; 52(65): 1347–1350.
4. Franson TR, Hierholzer WJ, Jr, and LaBrecque DR. Frequency and characteristics of hyperbilirubinemia associated with bacteremia. Rev Infect Dis 1985; 7(1): 1–9.
5. Szabo G, Romics L, Jr, and Frendl G. Liver in sepsis and systemic inflammatory response syndrome. Clin Liver Dis 2002; 6(4): 1045–1066, x.
6. Bolder U, Ton-Nu HT, Schteingart CD, Frick E, and Hofmann AF. Hepatocyte transport of bile acids and organic anions in endotoxemic rats: impaired uptake and secretion. Gastroenterology 1997; 112(1): 214–225.
7. Moseley RH. Sepsis-associated cholestasis. Gastroenterology 1997; 112(1): 302–306.
8. Green RM, Beier D, and Gollan JL. Regulation of hepatocyte bile salt transporters by endotoxin and inflammatory cytokines in rodents. Gastroenterology 1996; 111(1): 193–198.
9. Kubitz R, Wettstein M, Warskulat U, and Haussinger D. Regulation of the multidrug resistance protein 2 in the rat liver by lipopolysaccharide and dexamethasone. Gastroenterology 1999; 116(2): 401–410.
10. Lefkowitch JH. Bile ductular cholestasis: an ominous histopathologic sign related to sepsis and "cholangitis lenta". Hum Pathol 1982; 13(1): 19–24.
11. Lefkowitch JH. Histological assessment of cholestasis. Clin Liver Dis 2004; 8(1): 27–40, v.
12. Hirata K, Ikeda S, Honma T, et al. Sepsis and cholestasis: basic findings in the sinusoid and bile canaliculus. J Hepatobiliary Pancreat Surg 2001; 8(1): 20–26.
13. Kreek MJ. Female sex steroids and cholestasis. Semin Liver Dis 1987; 7(1): 8–23.
14. Kreek MJ and Sleisenger MH. Estrogen induced cholestasis due to endogenous and exogenous hormones. Scand J Gastroenterol Suppl 1970; 7: 123–131.
15. Vore M. Estrogen cholestasis. Membranes, metabolites, or receptors? Gastroenterology 1987; 93(3): 643–649.
16. Debry P, Nash EA, Neklason DW, and Metherall JE. Role of multidrug resistance P-glycoproteins in cholesterol esterification. J Biol Chem 1997; 272(2): 1026–1031.

17. Stieger B, Fattinger K, Madon J, Kullak-Ublick GA and Meier PJ. Drug- and estrogen-induced cholestasis through inhibition of the hepatocellular bile salt export pump (Bsep) of rat liver. Gastroenterology 2000; 118(2): 422–430.

18. Huang L, Smit JW, Meijer DK, and Vore M. Mrp2 is essential for estradiol-17beta (beta-D-glucuronide)-induced cholestasis in rats. Hepatology 2000; 32(1): 66–72.

19. Beuers U and Pusl T. Intrahepatic cholestasis of pregnancy—a heterogeneous group of pregnancy-related disorders? Hepatology 2006; 43(4): 647–649.

20. Rolfes DB and Ishak KG. Liver disease in pregnancy. Histopathology 1986; 10(6): 555–570.

21. Pauli-Magnus C, Lang T, Meier Y, et al. Sequence analysis of bile salt export pump (ABCB11) and multidrug resistance p-glycoprotein 3 (ABCB4, MDR3) in patients with intrahepatic cholestasis of pregnancy. Pharmacogenetics 2004; 14(2): 91–102.

22. Savander M, Ropponen A, Avela K, et al. Genetic evidence of heterogeneity in intrahepatic cholestasis of pregnancy. Gut 2003; 52(7): 1025–1029.

23. Mullenbach R, Linton KJ, Wiltshire S, et al. ABCB4 gene sequence variation in women with intrahepatic cholestasis of pregnancy. J Med Genet 2003; 40(5): e70.

24. Lucena JF, Herrero JI, Quiroga J, et al. A multidrug resistance 3 gene mutation causing cholelithiasis, cholestasis of pregnancy, and adulthood biliary cirrhosis. Gastroenterology 2003; 124(4): 1037–1042.

25. Jacquemin E, Cresteil D, Manouvrier S, Boute O, and Hadchouel M. Heterozygous non-sense mutation of the MDR3 gene in familial intrahepatic cholestasis of pregnancy. Lancet 1999; 353(9148): 210–211.

26. Mullenbach R, Bennett A, Tetlow N, et al. ATP8B1 mutations in British cases with intrahepatic cholestasis of pregnancy. Gut 2005; 54(6): 829–834.

27. Painter JN, Savander M, Ropponen A, et al. Sequence variation in the ATP8B1 gene and intrahepatic cholestasis of pregnancy. Eur J Hum Genet 2005; 13(4): 435–439.

28. Bacq Y, Sapey T, Brechot MC, Pierre F, Fignon A, and Dubois F. Intrahepatic cholestasis of pregnancy: a French prospective study. Hepatology 1997; 26(2): 358–364.

29. Ropponen A, Sund R, Riikonen S, Ylikorkala O, and Aittomaki K. Intrahepatic cholestasis of pregnancy as an indicator of liver and biliary diseases: a population-based study. Hepatology 2006; 43(4): 723–728.

30. Glantz A, Marschall HU, Lammert F, and Mattsson LA. Intrahepatic cholestasis of pregnancy: a randomized controlled trial comparing dexamethasone and ursodeoxycholic acid. Hepatology 2005; 42(6): 1399–1405.

31. Kondrackiene J, Beuers U, and Kupcinskas L. Efficacy and safety of ursodeoxycholic acid versus cholestyramine in intrahepatic cholestasis of pregnancy. Gastroenterology 2005; 129(3): 894–901.

32. Zapata R, Sandoval L, Palma J, et al. Ursodeoxycholic acid in the treatment of intrahepatic cholestasis of pregnancy. A 12-year experience. Liver Int 2005; 25(3): 548–554.

33. Roncaglia N, Locatelli A, Arreghini A, et al. A randomised controlled trial of ursodeoxycholic acid and S-adenosyl-L-methionine in the treatment of gestational cholestasis. Bjog 2004; 111(1): 17–21.

34. Nicastri PL, Diaferia A, Tartagni M, Loizzi P, and Fanelli M. A randomised placebo-controlled trial of ursodeoxycholic acid and S-adenosylmethionine in the treatment of intrahepatic cholestasis of pregnancy. Br J Obstet Gynaecol 1998; 105(11): 1205–1207.

35. Javitt NB. Cholestasis of pregnancy: ursodeoxycholic acid therapy. J Hepatol 1998; 29(5): 827–828.

36. Floreani A, Paternoster D, Melis A, and Grella PV. S-Adenosylmethionine versus ursodeoxycholic acid in the treatment of intrahepatic cholestasis of pregnancy: preliminary results of a controlled trial. Eur J Obstet Gynecol Reprod Biol 1996; 67(2): 109–113.

37. Diaferia A, Nicastri PL, Tartagni M, Loizzi P, Iacovizzi C, and Di Leo A. Ursodeoxycholic acid therapy in pregnant women with cholestasis. Int J Gynaecol Obstet 1996; 52(2): 133–140.

38. Davies MH, da Silva RC, Jones SR, Weaver JB, and Elias E. Fetal mortality associated with cholestasis of pregnancy and the potential benefit of therapy with ursodeoxycholic acid. Gut 1995; 37(4): 580–584.

39. Floreani A, Paternoster D, Grella V, Sacco S, Gangemi M, and Chiaramonte M. Ursodeoxycholic acid in intrahepatic cholestasis of pregnancy. Br J Obstet Gynaecol 1994; 101(1): 64–65.

40. Cogger VC, Fraser R, and Le Couteur DG. Liver dysfunction and heart failure. Am J Cardiol 2003; 91(11): 1399.

41. Moussavian SN, Dincsoy HP, Goodman S, Helm RA, and Bozian RC. Severe hyperbilirubinemia and coma in chronic congestive heart failure. Dig Dis Sci 1982; 27(2): 175–180.

42. Giallourakis CC, Rosenberg PM, and Friedman LS. The liver in heart failure. Clin Liver Dis 2002; 6(4): 947–967, viii–ix.

43. Lau GT, Tan HC, and Kritharides L. Type of liver dysfunction in heart failure and its relation to the severity of tricuspid regurgitation. Am J Cardiol 2002; 90(12): 1405–1409.

44. Batin P, Wickens M, McEntegart D, Fullwood L, and Cowley AJ. The importance of abnormalities of liver function tests in predicting mortality in chronic heart failure. Eur Heart J 1995; 16(11): 1613–1618.

45. Kubo SH, Walter BA, John DH, Clark M, and Cody RJ. Liver function abnormalities in chronic heart failure. Influence of systemic hemodynamics. Arch Intern Med 1987; 147(7): 1227–1230.

46. Richman SM, Delman AJ, and Grob D. Alterations in indices of liver function in congestive heart failure with particular reference to serum enzymes. Am J Med 1961; 30: 211–225.

47. Stauffer MH, Sauer WG, Dearing WH, and Baggenstoss AH. The spectrum of cholestatic hepatic disease. JAMA 1965; 191: 829–837.

48. Giannakos G, Papanicolaou X, Trafalis D, Michaelidis I, Margaritis G, and Christofilakis C. Stauffer's syndrome variant associated with renal cell carcinoma. Int J Urol 2005; 12(8): 757–759.

49. Dourakis SP, Sinani C, Deutsch M, Dimitriadou E, and Hadziyannis SJ. Cholestatic jaundice as a paraneoplastic manifestation of renal cell carcinoma. Eur J Gastroenterol Hepatol 1997; 9(3): 311–314.

50. Hanash KA. The nonmetastatic hepatic dysfunction syndrome associated with renal cell carcinoma (hypernephroma): Stauffer's syndrome. Prog Clin Biol Res 1982; 100: 301–316.

51. Delpre G, Ilie B, Papo J, Streifler C, and Gefel A. Hypernephroma with non-metastatic liver dysfunction (Stauffer's syndrome) and hypercalcemia. Case report and review of the literature. Am J Gastroenterol 1979; 72(3): 239–247.

52. Jacobi GH and Philipp T. Stauffer's syndrome—diagnostic help in hypernephroma. Clin Nephrol 1975; 4(3): 113–115.

53. Andrassy K, Gartner H, Siede WH, et al. Stauffer's syndrome in renal cell carcinoma evidence for intravascular coagulation. Klin Wochenschr 1980; 58(2): 91–97.

54. Aoyagi T, Mori I, Ueyama Y, and Tamaoki N. Sinusoidal dilatation of the liver as a paraneoplastic manifestation of renal cell carcinoma. Hum Pathol 1989; 20(12): 1193–1197.
55. Karakolios A, Kasapis C, Kallinikidis T, Kalpidis P, and Grigoriadis N. Cholestatic jaundice as a paraneoplastic manifestation of prostate adenocarcinoma. Clin Gastroenterol Hepatol 2003; 1(6): 480–483.
56. Blay JY, Rossi JF, Wijdenes J, et al. Role of interleukin-6 in the paraneoplastic inflammatory syndrome associated with renal-cell carcinoma. Int J Cancer 1997; 72(3): 424–430.
57. Walther MM, Johnson B, Culley D, et al. Serum interleukin-6 levels in metastatic renal cell carcinoma before treatment with interleukin-2 correlates with paraneoplastic syndromes but not patient survival. J Urol 1998; 159(3): 718–722.
58. Chung CH, Wang CH, Tzen CY, and Liu CP. Intrahepatic cholestasis as a paraneoplastic syndrome associated with pheochromocytoma. J Endocrinol Invest 2005; 28(2): 175–179.
59. Green RM, Whiting JF, Rosenbluth AB, Beier D, and Gollan JL. Interleukin-6 inhibits hepatocyte taurocholate uptake and sodium-potassium-adenosinetriphosphatase activity. Am J Physiol 1994; 267(6 Pt 1): G1094–G1100.
60. Denson LA, Auld KL, Schiek DS, McClure MH, Mangelsdorf DJ, and Karpen SJ. Interleukin-1beta suppresses retinoid transactivation of two hepatic transporter genes involved in bile formation. J Biol Chem 2000; 275(12): 8835–8843.
61. Jakobovits AW, Crimmins FB, Sherlock S, Erlinger S, and Rambaud J. Cholestasis as a paraneoplastic manifestation of carcinoma of the kidney. Aust N Z J Med 1981; 11(1): 64–67.
62. Koruk M, Buyukberber M, Savas C, and Kadayifci A. Paraneoplastic cholestasis associated with prostate carcinoma. Turk J Gastroenterol 2004; 15(1): 53–55.
63. Tiede DJ, Tefferi A, Kochhar R, Thompson GB, and Hay ID. Paraneoplastic cholestasis and hypercoagulability associated with medullary thyroid carcinoma. Resolution with tumor debulking. Cancer 1994; 73(3): 702–705.
64. Safyan EL, Veerabagu MP, Swerdlow SH, Lee RG, and Rakela J. Intrahepatic cholestasis due to systemic mastocytosis: a case report and review of literature. Am J Gastroenterol 1997; 92(7): 1197–1200.
65. Jones AL, Schmucker DL, Renston RH, and Murakami T. The architecture of bile secretion. A morphological perspective of physiology. Dig Dis Sci 1980; 25(8): 609–629.
66. Cox CE, Davis-Allen A, and Judson MA. Sarcoidosis. Med Clin North Am 2005; 89(4): 817–828.
67. Matheus T and Munoz S. Granulomatous liver disease and cholestasis. Clin Liver Dis 2004; 8(1): 229–246, ix.
68. Denk H, Scheuer PJ, Baptista A, et al. Guidelines for the diagnosis and interpretation of hepatic granulomas. Histopathology 1994; 25(3): 209–218.
69. Bolukbas C, Bolukbas FF, Kebdir T, et al. Development of sarcoidosis during interferon alpha 2b and ribavirin combination therapy for chronic hepatitis C—a case report and review of the literature. Acta Gastroenterol Belg 2005; 68(4): 432–434.
70. Hunt J, Gordon FD, Jenkins RL, Lewis WD, and Khettry U. Sarcoidosis with selective involvement of a second liver allograft: report of a case and review of the literature. Mod Pathol 1999; 12(3): 325–328.
71. Klatskin G and Yesner R. Hepatic manifestations of sarcoidosis and other granulomatous diseases; a study based on histological examination of tissue obtained by needle biopsy of the liver. Yale J Biol Med 1950; 23(3): 207–248.

72. Shay H, Berk JE, Sones M, Aegerter EE, Weston JK, and Adams AB. The liver in sarcoidosis. Gastroenterology 1951; 19(3): 441–461.
73. Branson JH and Park JH. Sarcoidosishepatic involvement: presentation of a case with fatal liver involvement; including autopsy findings and review of the evidence for sarcoid involvement of the liver as found in the literature. Ann Intern Med 1954; 40(1): 111–145.
74. Devaney K, Goodman ZD, Epstein MS, Zimmerman HJ, and Ishak KG. Hepatic sarcoidosis. Clinicopathologic features in 100 patients. Am J Surg Pathol 1993; 17(12): 1272–1280.
75. Blich M and Edoute Y. Clinical manifestations of sarcoid liver disease. J Gastroenterol Hepatol 2004; 19(7): 732–737.
76. Bilir M, Mert A, Ozaras R, et al. Hepatic sarcoidosis: clinicopathologic features in thirty-seven patients. J Clin Gastroenterol 2000; 31(4): 337–338.
77. James DG and Sherlock S. Sarcoidosis of the liver. Sarcoidosis 1994; 11(1): 2–6.
78. Ishak KG. Sarcoidosis of the liver and bile ducts. Mayo Clin Proc 1998; 73(5): 467–472.
79. Alam I, Levenson SD, Ferrell LD, and Bass NM. Diffuse intrahepatic biliary strictures in sarcoidosis resembling sclerosing cholangitis. Case report and review of the literature. Dig Dis Sci 1997; 42(6): 1295–1301.
80. Rezeig MA and Fashir BM. Biliary tract obstruction due to sarcoidosis: a case report. Am J Gastroenterol 1997; 92(3): 527–528.
81. Russi EW, Bansky G, Pfaltz M, Spinas G, Hammer B, and Senning A. Budd-Chiari syndrome in sarcoidosis. Am J Gastroenterol 1986; 81(1): 71–75.
82. Nataline MR, Goyette RE, Owensby LC, and Rubin RN. The Budd-Chiari syndrome in sarcoidosis. JAMA 1978; 239(25): 2657.
83. Nakanuma Y, Kouda W, Harada K, and Hiramatsu K. Hepatic sarcoidosis with vanishing bile duct syndrome, cirrhosis, and portal phlebosclerosis. Report of an autopsy case. J Clin Gastroenterol 2001; 32(2): 181–184.
84. Moreno-Merlo F, Wanless IR, Shimamatsu K, Sherman M, Greig P, and Chiasson D. The role of granulomatous phlebitis and thrombosis in the pathogenesis of cirrhosis and portal hypertension in sarcoidosis. Hepatology 1997; 26(3): 554–560.
85. Salazar A, Mana J, Sala J, Landoni BR, and Manresa F. Combined portal and pulmonary hypertension in sarcoidosis. Respiration 1994; 61(2): 117–119.
86. Bass NM, Burroughs AK, Scheuer PJ, James DG, and Sherlock S. Chronic intrahepatic cholestasis due to sarcoidosis. Gut 1982; 23(5): 417–421.
87. Berger I and Katz M. Portal hypertension due to hepatic sarcoidosis. Am J Gastroenterol 1973; 59(2): 147–151.
88. Amarapurkar DN, Patel ND, and Amarapurkar AD. Hepatic sarcoidosis. Indian J Gastroenterol 2003; 22(3): 98–100.
89. Melissant CF, Smith SJ, Kazzaz BA, and Demedts M. Bleeding varices due to portal hypertension in sarcoidosis. Favorable effect of propranolol and prednisone. Chest 1993; 103(2): 628–629.
90. Gerard AG, Roth AL, Becker SM, and Shih CS. Regression of sarcoid hepatosplenomegaly on corticosteroid therapy. J Med Soc N J 1968; 65(2): 64–67.
91. Valla D, Pessegueiro-Miranda H, Degott C, Lebrec D, Rueff B, and Benhamou JP. Hepatic sarcoidosis with portal hypertension. A report of seven cases with a review of the literature. QJM 1987; 63(242): 531–544.
92. Vatti R and Sharma OP. Course of asymptomatic liver involvement in sarcoidosis: role of therapy in selected cases. Sarcoidosis Vasc. Diffuse Lung Dis 1997; 14(1): 73–76.

93. Becheur H, Dall'osto H, Chatellier G, et al. Effect of ursodeoxycholic acid on chronic intrahepatic cholestasis due to sarcoidosis. Dig Dis Sci 1997; 42(4): 789–791.
94. Hughes GS, Jr, Kataria YP, and O'Brien TF, Jr. Sarcoidosis presenting as biliary cirrhosis: treatment with chlorambucil. South Med J 1983; 76(11): 1440–1442.
95. Galwankar S, Vyas M, Desai D, and Udwadia ZF. Hepatic sarcoidosis responding to chloroquine as steroid-sparing drug. Indian J Gastroenterol 1999; 18(4): 177–178.
96. Cengiz C, Rodriguez-Davalos M, deBoccardo G, et al. Recurrent hepatic sarcoidosis post-liver transplantation manifesting with severe hypercalcemia: a case report and review of the literature. Liver Transpl 2005; 11(12): 1611–1614.
97. Lipson EJ, Fiel MI, Florman SS, and Korenblat KM. Patient and graft outcomes following liver transplantation for sarcoidosis. Clin Transplant 2005; 19(4): 487–491.
98. Shibolet O, Kalish Y, Wolf D, et al. Exacerbation of pulmonary sarcoidosis after liver transplantation. J Clin Gastroenterol 2002; 35(4): 356–358.
99. Fidler HM, Hadziyannis SJ, Dhillon AP, Sherlock S, and Burroughs AK. Recurrent hepatic sarcoidosis following liver transplantation. Transplant Proc 1997; 29(5): 2509–2510.
100. Kinnman N, Lindblad A, Housset C, et al. Expression of cystic fibrosis transmembrane conductance regulator in liver tissue from patients with cystic fibrosis. Hepatology 2000; 32(2): 334–340.
101. Bass S, Connon JJ, and Ho CS. Biliary tree in cystic fibrosis. Biliary tract abnormalities in cystic fibrosis demonstrated by endoscopic retrograde cholangiography. Gastroenterology 1983; 84(6): 1592–1596.
102. Colombo C, Apostolo MG, Assaisso M, Roman B, and Bottani P. Liver disease in cystic fibrosis. Neth J Med 1992; 41(3–4): 119–122.
103. Roy CC, Weber AM, Morin CL, et al. Hepatobiliary disease in cystic fibrosis: a survey of current issues and concepts. J Pediatr Gastroenterol Nutr 1982; 1(4): 469–478.
104. Vawter GF and Shwachman H. Cystic fibrosis in adults: an autopsy study. Pathol. Annu. 1979; 14 (Pt 2): 357–382.
105. Colombo C, Battezzati PM, Crosignani A, et al. Liver disease in cystic fibrosis: A prospective study on incidence, risk factors, and outcome. Hepatology 2002; 36(6): 1374–1382.
106. Lindblad A, Glaumann H, and Strandvik B. Natural history of liver disease in cystic fibrosis. Hepatology 1999; 30(5): 1151–1158.
107. Lamireau T, Monnereau S, Martin S, Marcotte JE, Winnock M, and Alvarez F. Epidemiology of liver disease in cystic fibrosis: a longitudinal study. J Hepatol 2004; 41(6): 920–925.
108. Cheng K, Ashby D, and Smyth R. Ursodeoxycholic acid for cystic fibrosis-related liver disease. Cochrane Database Syst Rev 2000; (2): CD000222.
109. Colombo C, Battezzati PM, Podda M, Bettinardi N, and Giunta A. Ursodeoxycholic acid for liver disease associated with cystic fibrosis: a double-blind multicenter trial. The Italian Group for the Study of Ursodeoxycholic Acid in Cystic Fibrosis. Hepatology 1996; 23(6): 1484–1490.
110. Colombo C, Crosignani A, Assaisso M, et al. Ursodeoxycholic acid therapy in cystic fibrosis-associated liver disease: a dose-response study. Hepatology 1992; 16(4): 924–930.
111. Cotting J, Lentze MJ, and Reichen J. Effects of ursodeoxycholic acid treatment on nutrition and liver function in patients with cystic fibrosis and longstanding cholestasis. Gut 1990; 31(8): 918–921.

112. Galabert C, Montet JC, Lengrand D, et al. Effects of ursodeoxycholic acid on liver function in patients with cystic fibrosis and chronic cholestasis. J Pediatr 1992; 121(1): 138–141.

113. Lindblad A, Glaumann H, and Strandvik B. A two-year prospective study of the effect of ursodeoxycholic acid on urinary bile acid excretion and liver morphology in cystic fibrosis-associated liver disease. Hepatology 1998; 27(1): 166–174.

114. Nousia-Arvanitakis S, Fotoulaki M, Economou H, Xefteri M, and Galli-Tsinopoulou A. Long-term prospective study of the effect of ursodeoxycholic acid on cystic fibrosis-related liver disease. J Clin Gastroenterol 2001; 32(4): 324–328.

115. Molmenti EP, Squires RH, Nagata D, et al. Liver transplantation for cholestasis associated with cystic fibrosis in the pediatric population. Pediatr Transplant 2003; 7(2): 93–97.

116. Jonas MM. The role of liver transplantation in cystic fibrosis re-examined. Liver Transpl 2005; 11(12): 1463–1465.

117. Gooding I, Dondos V, Gyi KM, Hodson M, and Westaby D. Variceal hemorrhage and cystic fibrosis: outcomes and implications for liver transplantation. Liver Transpl 2005; 11(12): 1522–1526.

118. von Knorring J and Wassatjerna C. Liver involvement in polymyalgia rheumatica. Scand J Rheumatol 1976; 5(4): 197–204.

119. Abraham S, Begum S, and Isenberg D. Hepatic manifestations of autoimmune rheumatic diseases. Ann Rheum Dis 2004; 63(2): 123–129.

120. Webb J, Whaley K, MacSween RN, Nuki G, Dick WC, and Buchanan WW. Liver disease in rheumatoid arthritis and Sjogren's syndrome. Prospective study using biochemical and serological markers of hepatic dysfunction. Ann Rheum Dis 1975; 34(1): 70–81.

121. Cockel R, Kendall MJ, Becker JF, and Hawkins CF. Serum biochemical values in rheumatoid disease. Ann Rheum Dis 1971; 30(2): 166–170.

122. Kendall MJ, Cockel R, Becker J, and Hawkins CF. Raised serum alkaline phosphatase in rheumatoid disease. An index of liver dysfunction? Ann Rheum Dis 1970; 29(5): 537–540.

123. Fernandes L, Sullivan S, McFarlane IG, et al. Studies on the frequency and pathogenesis of liver involvement in rheumatoid arthritis. Ann Rheum Dis 1979; 38(6): 501–506.

124. Blendis LM, Ansell ID, Jones KL, Hamilton E, and Williams R. Liver in Felty's syndrome. BMJ 1970; 1(689): 131–135.

125. Thorne C, Urowitz MB, Wanless I, Roberts E, and Blendis LM. Liver disease in Felty's syndrome. Am J Med 1982; 73(1): 35–40.

126. Rau R, Pfenninger K, and Boni A. Proceedings: Liver function tests and liver biopsies in patients with rheumatoid arthritis. Ann Rheum Dis 1975; 34(2): 198–199.

127. Clarke AK, Galbraith RM, Hamilton EB, and Williams R. Rheumatic disorders in primary biliary cirrhosis. Ann Rheum Dis 1978; 37(1): 42–47.

128. Zukowski TH, Jorgensen RA, Dickson ER, and Lindor KD. Autoimmune conditions associated with primary biliary cirrhosis: response to ursodeoxycholic acid therapy. Am J Gastroenterol 1998; 93(6): 958–961.

129. Farre JM, Perez T, Hautefeuille P, et al. Cholestasis and pneumonitis induced by gold therapy. Clin Rheumatol 1989; 8(4): 538–540.

130. Hanissian AS, Rothschild BM, and Kaplan S. Gold: hepatotoxic and cholestatic reactions. Clin Rheumatol 1985; 4(2): 183–188.

131. Basset C, Vadrot J, Denis J, Poupon J, and Zafrani ES. Prolonged cholestasis and ductopenia following gold salt therapy. Liver Int 2003; 23(2): 89–93.

132. Multz CV. Cholestatic hepatitis caused by penicillamine. JAMA 1981; 246(6): 674–675.

133. Barzilai D, Dickstein G, Enat R, Bassan H, Lichtig C, and Gellei B. Cholestatic jaundice caused by D-penicillamine. Ann Rheum Dis 1978; 37(1): 98–100.

134. Mitrane MP, Singh A, and Seibold JR. Cholestasis and fatal agranulocytosis complicating sulfasalazine therapy: case report and review of the literature. J Rheumatol 1986; 13(5): 969–972.

135. Cavalli G, Casali AM, Lambertini F, and Busachi C. Changes in the small biliary passages in the hepatic localization of Hodgkin's disease. Virchows Arch. A Pathol Anat Histol 1979; 384(3): 295–306.

136. Lefkowitch JH, Falkow S, and Whitlock RT. Hepatic Hodgkin's disease simulating cholestatic hepatitis with liver failure. Arch Pathol Lab Med 1985; 109(5): 424–426.

137. Trotter MC, Cloud GA, Davis M, et al. Predicting the risk of abdominal disease in Hodgkin's lymphoma. A multifactorial analysis of staging laparotomy results in 255 patients. Ann Surg 1985; 201(4): 465–469.

138. Sans M, Andreu V, Bordas JM, et al. Usefulness of laparoscopy with liver biopsy in the assessment of liver involvement at diagnosis of Hodgkin's and non-Hodgkin's lymphomas. Gastrointest Endosc 1998; 47(5): 391–395.

139. Abt AB, Kirschner RH, Belliveau RE, et al. Hepatic pathology associated with Hodgkin's disease. Cancer 1974; 33(6): 1564–1571.

140. Lotz MJ, Chabner B, DeVita VT Jr, Johnson RE, and Berard CW. Pathological staging of 100 consecutive untreated patients with non-Hodgkin's lymphomas: extramedullary sites of disease. Cancer 1976; 37(1): 266–270.

141. Roth A, Kolaric K, and Dominis M. Histologic and cytologic liver changes in 120 patients with malignant lymphomas. Tumori 1978; 64(1): 45–53.

142. de Medeiros BC, Lacerda MA, Telles JE, da Silva JA, and de Medeiros CR. Cholestasis secondary to Hodgkin's disease: report of 2 cases of vanishing bile duct syndrome. Haematologica 1998; 83(11): 1038–1040.

143. Gottrand F, Cullu F, Mazingue F, Nelken B, Lecomte-Houcke M, and Farriaux JP. Intrahepatic cholestasis related to vanishing bile duct syndrome in Hodgkin's disease. J Pediatr Gastroenterol Nutr 1997; 24(4): 430–433.

144. Yalcin S, Kars A, Sokmensuer C, and Atahan L. Extrahepatic Hodgkin's disease with intrahepatic cholestasis: report of two cases. Oncology 1999; 57(1): 83–85.

145. Perera DR, Greene ML, and Fenster LF. Cholestasis associated with extrabiliary Hodgkin's disease. Report of three cases and review of four others. Gastro-enterology 1974; 67(4): 680–685.

146. Lieberman DA. Intrahepatic cholestasis due to Hodgkin's disease. An elusive diagnosis. J Clin Gastroenterol 1986; 8(3 Pt 1): 304–307.

147. Liangpunsakul S, Kwo P, and Koukoulis GK. Hodgkin's disease presenting as cholestatic hepatitis with prominent ductal injury. Eur J Gastroenterol Hepatol 2002; 14(3): 323–327.

148. Hubscher SG, Lumley MA, and Elias E. Vanishing bile duct syndrome: a possible mechanism for intrahepatic cholestasis in Hodgkin's lymphoma. Hepatology 1993; 17(1): 70–77.

149. Abe H, Kubota K, and Makuuchi M. Obstructive jaundice secondary to Hodgkin's disease. Am J Gastroenterol 1997; 92(3): 526–527.

150. Fidias P, Carey RW, and Grossbard ML. Non-Hodgkin's lymphoma presenting with biliary tract obstruction. A discussion of seven patients and a review of the literature. Cancer 1995; 75(7): 1669–1677.
151. Salmon JS, Thompson MA, Arildsen RC, and Greer JP. Non-Hodgkin's lymphoma involving the liver: clinical and therapeutic considerations. Clin Lymphoma Myeloma 2006; 6(4): 273–280.
152. Rowbotham D, Wendon J, and Williams R. Acute liver failure secondary to hepatic infiltration: a single centre experience of 18 cases. Gut 1998; 42(4): 576–580.
153. Braude S, Gimson AE, Portmann B, and Williams R. Fulminant hepatic failure in non-Hodgkin's lymphoma. Postgrad Med J 1982; 58(679): 301–304.
154. Murai M, Yoneyama H, Harada A, et al. Active participation of CCR5(+)CD8(+) T lymphocytes in the pathogenesis of liver injury in graft-versus-host disease. J Clin Invest 1999; 104(1): 49–57.
155. Shulman HM, Sharma P, Amos D, Fenster LF, and McDonald GB. A coded histologic study of hepatic graft-versus-host disease after human bone marrow transplantation. Hepatology 1988; 8(3): 463–470.
156. Deeg HJ and Storb R. Graft-versus-host disease: pathophysiological and clinical aspects. Annu Rev Med 1984; 35: 11–24.
157. Ma SY, Au WY, Ng IO, et al. Hepatitic graft-versus-host disease after hematopoietic stem cell transplantation: clinicopathologic features and prognostic implication. Transplantation 2004; 77(8): 1252–1259.
158. Hogan WJ, Maris M, Storer B, et al. Hepatic injury after nonmyeloablative conditioning followed by allogeneic hematopoietic cell transplantation: a study of 193 patients. Blood 2004; 103(1): 78–84.
159. Fujii N, Takenaka K, Shinagawa K, et al. Hepatic graft-versus-host disease presenting as an acute hepatitis after allogeneic peripheral blood stem cell transplantation. Bone Marrow Transplant 2001; 27(9): 1007–1010.
160. Schwinghammer TL and Bloom EJ. Pharmacologic prophylaxis of acute graft-versus-host disease after allogeneic marrow transplantation. Clin Pharm 1993; 12(10): 736–761.
161. Ratanatharathorn V, Ayash L, Lazarus HM, Fu J, and Uberti JP. Chronic graft-versus-host disease: clinical manifestation and therapy. Bone Marrow Transplant 2001; 28(2): 121–129.
162. Knapp AB, Crawford JM, Rappeport JM, and Gollan JL. Cirrhosis as a consequence of graft-versus-host disease. Gastroenterology 1987; 92(2): 513–519.
163. Siegert W, Stemerowicz R, and Hopf U. Antimitochondrial antibodies in patients with chronic graft-versus-host disease. Bone Marrow Transplant 1992; 10(3): 221–227.
164. Quaranta S, Shulman H, Ahmed A, et al. Autoantibodies in human chronic graft-versus-host disease after hematopoietic cell transplantation. Clin Immunol 1999; 91(1): 106–116.
165. Fried RH, Murakami CS, Fisher LD, Willson RA, Sullivan KM, and McDonald GB. Ursodeoxycholic acid treatment of refractory chronic graft-versus-host disease of the liver. Ann Intern Med 1992; 116(8): 624–629.
166. Pavletic SZ, Smith LM, Bishop MR, et al. Prognostic factors of chronic graft-versus-host disease after allogeneic blood stem-cell transplantation. Am J Hematol 2005; 78(4): 265–274.
167. Kumar S, Chen MG, Gastineau DA, et al. Prophylaxis of graft-versus-host disease with cyclosporine-prednisone is associated with increased risk of chronic graft-versus-host disease. Bone Marrow Transplant 2001; 27(11): 1133–1140.

168. Strasser SI, Sullivan KM, Myerson D, et al. Cirrhosis of the liver in long-term marrow transplant survivors. Blood 1999; 93(10): 3259–3266.
169. Teixidor HS, Godwin TA, and Ramirez EA. Cryptosporidiosis of the biliary tract in AIDS. Radiology 1991; 180(1): 51–56.
170. Teixidor HS, Honig CL, Norsoph E, Albert S, Mouradian JA, and Whalen JP. Cytomegalovirus infection of the alimentary canal: radiologic findings with pathologic correlation. Radiology 1987; 163(2): 317–323.
171. Benhamou Y, Caumes E, Gerosa Y, et al. AIDS-related cholangiopathy. Critical analysis of a prospective series of 26 patients. Dig Dis Sci 1993; 38(6): 1113–1118.
172. Cello JP. Acquired immunodeficiency syndrome cholangiopathy: spectrum of disease. Am J Med 1989; 86(5): 539–546.
173. Mahajani RV and Uzer MF. Cholangiopathy in HIV-infected patients. Clin Liver Dis 1999; 3(3): 669–684, x.
174. Hohn DC, Stagg RJ, Friedman MA, et al. A randomized trial of continuous intravenous versus hepatic intraarterial floxuridine in patients with colorectal cancer metastatic to the liver: the Northern California Oncology Group trial. J Clin Oncol 1989; 7(11): 1646–1654.
175. Doria MI, Jr, Shepard KV, Levin B, and Riddell RH. Liver pathology following hepatic arterial infusion chemotherapy. Hepatic toxicity with FUDR. Cancer 1986; 58(4): 855–861.
176. Kemeny MM, Battifora H, Blayney DW, et al. Sclerosing cholangitis after continuous hepatic artery infusion of FUDR. Ann Surg 1985; 202(2): 176–181.
177. Ludwig J, Kim CH, Wiesner RH, and Krom RA. Floxuridine-induced sclerosing cholangitis: an ischemic cholangiopathy? Hepatology 1989; 9(2): 215–218.
178. Aldrighetti L, Arru M, Ronzoni M, Salvioni M, Villa E, and Ferla G. Extrahepatic biliary stenoses after hepatic arterial infusion (HAI) of floxuridine (FUdR) for liver metastases from colorectal cancer. Hepatogastroenterology 2001; 48(41): 1302–1307.
179. Pien EH, Zeman RK, Benjamin SB, et al. Iatrogenic sclerosing cholangitis following hepatic arterial chemotherapy infusion. Radiology 1985; 156(2): 329–330.
180. Mohi-ud-din R and Lewis JH. Drug- and chemical-induced cholestasis. Clin Liver Dis 2004; 8(1): 95–132, vii.

9 Complications of Cholestasis

Abhitabh Patil and Marlyn J. Mayo

CONTENTS

Abstract

It is important to recognize the complications of cholestasis in patients with chronic cholestatic liver disease because of their prevalence and their pre- and post-transplant implications. Understanding and treating these conditions can result in a significant impact on morbidity and quality of life in this group of patients. Most of what is known is based on small studies of patients with primary biliary cirrhosis (PBC) and primary sclerosing cholangitis (PSC), which is then extrapolated to patients with other cholestatic diseases. This section will review the pathophysiology and management of osteoporosis, pruritus, dyslipidemia, and vitamin deficiencies.

Key Words: Cholestasis; pruritus; osteoporosis; vitamin deficiency; dyslipidemia.

1. OSTEOPOROSIS

1.1. Prevalence

Osteoporosis occurs in cirrhosis of all etiologies, not just cholestatic liver disease *(1)*. The severity of osteoporosis varies according to the type, severity, and progression of the underlying liver disease. The prevalence of osteoporosis in end-stage primary biliary cirrhosis (PBC)

From: *Clinical Gastroenterology: Cholestatic Liver Disease*
Edited by: K. D. Lindor and J. A. Talwalkar © Humana Press Inc., Totowa, NJ

patients is 41% with fractures occurring in 21% of these patients *(2)*. Similarly, the prevalence of osteoporosis in primary sclerosing cholangitis (PSC) is 32% with fractures occurring in 16% of these patients *(3)*. The prevalence of osteoporosis is higher in patients with stage III and IV disease than stage I and II disease *(2–4)*. Children with chronic cholestasis also develop osteopenia proportional to disease severity and progression *(5)*.

Following liver transplantation, there is a rapid loss of bone during the first 3–6 months, which is believed to be related to the immunosuppressive medications and catabolic state in the peri-transplantation period *(6)*. Sometime during the first 4 mo, bone formation rates begin to increase; but they do not overtake the increased rate of bone resorption *(4)* until approximately 12–24 months post-transplantation, when a gradual increase in total bone mass is noted *(6)*. The incidence of post-transplant fractures is as high as 30–40% in cholestatic patients *(7)*. Patients at highest risk for post-transplant complications are those with a low pre-transplant bone mineral density (BMD) and a previous history of fracture. Thus, it is imperative to identify and aggressively manage osteopenia and osteoporosis in pre-transplant patients with chronic cholestatic liver disease.

1.2. Pathophysiology

Osteoporosis in cholestatic patients is believed to be multifactorial. Older age, higher Mayo risk score, lower body mass index, and advanced histological stage are all independent risk factors for osteoporosis in PBC patients *(8)*. Although menopausal status is the most common risk factor for osteoporosis in the general population, it does not confer a measurable added risk of osteoporosis to the factors listed above in PBC patients *(8)*.

Both increased resorption and decreased formation of bone contribute to the development of osteoporosis in cholestatic patients *(9)*. Although levels of 25-OH vitamin D are low in these patients, the ability to hydroxylate vitamin D *(10)* and hence the level of 1,25-OH2 vitamin D *(11)* are usually normal. The level of 25-OH vitamin D can rapidly be corrected with oral supplementation *(12)*; however, osteoporosis still progresses *(13)*. Moreover, calcium and vitamin D supplementation, even in the presence of vitamin D deficiency, does not reliably improve lumbar spine BMD in patients with PBC *(14)*. Thus, bone disease in cholestatic patients is not likely solely because of 25-hydroxylate or 1,25-hydroxylate vitamin D deficiency *(11)*.

Specific polymorphisms of the vitamin D receptor (BsmI BB genotype) and estrogen receptor alpha (PvuII and XbaIPp) are found more frequently in patients with PBC. However, no association has been found with BMD, bone mass, or risk of vertebral fracture *(15,16)*. Thus, it is unlikely that these polymorphisms are instrumental in the pathogenesis of BMD in these patients.

Osteocalcin, a protein thought to promote normal bone mineralization, is synthesized by osteoblasts and is dependent on vitamin K for its γ-carboxylation. Osteocalcin-knockout mice develop severe osteopenia. Thus, vitamin K has been proposed as a potential therapy for cholestatic osteoporosis. Vitamin K supplementation enhances osteocalcin accumulation in the extracellular matrix of osteoblasts *(17)*. It also inhibits osteoclast differentiation and induces osteoclast apoptosis *(18)*. Vitamin K therapy also slows the progression of bone loss seen in cholestatic patients *(19,20)*.

Unconjugated bilirubin may have a direct impact on bone metabolism. Patients with cholestatic liver disease have low markers of osteoblastic activity when compared to the normal population. When serum from these patients is added to that of normal patients, markers of osteoblastic activity also decrease. This effect is dose dependent. If the serum from cholestatic patients is photobleached, a process whereby unconjugated bilirubin is removed from the plasma, the effect on osteoblastic activity is abrogated *(21)*. Therefore, bilirubin probably has a direct, negative impact on osteoblastic activity, which may account for part of the correlation between the severity of cholestatic liver disease and the degree of osteoporosis.

1.3. Therapy

There are no randomized controlled trials sufficiently powered to demonstrate the prevention of fractures in cholestatic liver disease with therapy. Published recommendations are based on changes in BMD alone as a marker of efficacy and, thus, should be taken with prudence (Table 1). The American Association for the Study of Liver Diseases recommends beginning screening for osteoporosis in PBC patients at the time of diagnosis of cholestatic liver disease and repeating BMD exams every 1–2 yrs. Treatment can then be initiated if T-score $\leq$–2.5, Z-score $\leq$–1.5, or as clinically indicated.

The National Institute of Health guidelines suggest calcium supplementation of 1000 mg/d for all adults and 1500 mg/d for those at risk for osteoporosis and vitamin D supplementation of 800 IU/d for all adults and 50,000 IU given 2–3 times per week for those found to be deficient or at risk for osteoporosis. Although the ability of calcium and vitamin D supplementation to prevent deterioration of BMD in cholestatic

Table 1
Treatment Options for Osteoporosis

Calcium 1500 mg/d
Alendronate 70 mg/wk
Hormone replacement therapy various*
Fluoride 50 mg/d
Vitamin K (phytonadione) 1 mg/d

*Transdermal estradiol 50 μg/d two times per week+
medroxyprogesterone 2.5 mg/d; other regimens have been
studied and are presumed to be equally efficacious.

patients with osteoporosis has not been clearly demonstrated, it is safe, inexpensive, and reasonable to use as a preventative measure.

Estrogen supplementation is safe and effective for long-term use in cholestatic patients in improving total body BMD without causing significant changes in the liver function tests *(14,22,23)*. Newer agents useful in the treatment of conventional osteoporosis have yet to be proven effective in cholestatic patients with bone disease. Specifically, further studies are needed with respect to selective estrogen receptor modulators. In the MORE trial in noncholestatic, postmenopausal women with osteoporosis, raloxifene (a selective estrogen receptor modulator) in combination with calcium and cholecalciferol increased BMD in the spine and femoral neck and reduced the risk of vertebral fracture *(24)*. Raloxifene has been tested in a pilot study of nine PBC subjects with promising improvements in BMD *(25)*. Selective estrogen receptor modulating agents may eventually have a role in cholestatic patients, but further studies targeting cholestatic patients are needed.

Sodium fluoride stimulates bone formation, and it prevented bone loss in a 2-year, prospective, double-blind trial of PBC patients *(26)*. Though very effective at preventing bone loss and reducing the risk of fractures, side effects of severe dyspepsia limit its use. One randomized trial compared cyclical etidronate, a bisphosphonate, to fluoride and showed etidronate to be better tolerated and more effective than fluoride at preventing bone loss in PBC *(27)*. However, a subsequent randomized controlled trial of etidronate in PBC subjects with established osteopenia (T-score <-2.0) found that etidronate was no more effective than placebo *(28)*.

Alendronate, another bisphosphonate, effectively increases bone mass and has a greater antiresorptive power when compared to etidronate and is associated with minor to no side effects *(29,30)*. The theoretical risk of inducing variceal hemorrhage has not been shown to occur in clinical studies involving 33 patients with PBC.

There are several medications available for the treatment of postmenopausal osteoporosis which have not shown efficacy in trials of cholestatic patients. For example, parenterally administered calcitonin did not stop the progression of bone disease in a cohort of PBC subjects *(31)*. Another study evaluating subcutaneous calcitonin therapy given during the first 6 mo after liver transplantation showed that calcitonin did not prevent or reduce accelerated bone loss or spontaneous fractures *(32)*. Though there are trials showing benefit from PTH in patients with postmenopausal osteoporosis, *(33)* there are no trials with PTH in patients with cholestatic liver disease.

Vitamin K derivatives, phytonadione and menaquinone, may be quite effective for the prevention and treatment of osteoporosis resulting from cholestasis *(34)*. A randomized, control trial showed a higher BMD in patients receiving vitamin K when compared to placebo *(35)*. Given the low incidence of side effects and demonstrated efficacy, vitamin K should be considered as part of osteoporosis treatment in cholestatic liver disease.

2. PRURITUS

2.1. Prevalence

Pruritus is a common presenting symptom of cholestatic liver disease and affects nearly 70% of PBC patients within 10 years of diagnosis *(36)*.

2.2. Pathophysiology

The mechanism of cholestatic pruritus is poorly understood. The observed phenomenon of inducing pruritus via instillation of bile salts led to the theory that the retention and subsequent deposition of bile salts induces pruritus *(37)*. Unlike allergic pruritus, studies do not support the role of histamine in cholestatic pruritus. There is no difference in mast cell density, neural density, or the interaction between mast cells and neural cells in patients with cholestatic liver disease and normal patients *(38)*. This may explain the clinical observation that agents such as antihistamines and capsaicin are largely ineffective in cholestatic pruritus. More recently, opioid peptides in the CNS have been proposed as important mediators in the perception of itch in cholestatic patients *(39)*. Centrally administered opioid agonists in animal studies induce generalized pruritus *(40)*. Patients with cholestatic liver disease have increased plasma concentrations of endogenous opioid peptides,

Table 2
Treatment Options for Pruritus

Cholestyramine 4–16 g/d
Rifampin 300–600 mg/d
Nalmefene 4–240 mg/d
Naloxone 4 mg i.v., then 0.2 μg min/kg
Naltrexone 50 mg/d
Sertraline 75–100 mg/d

methionine enkephalin and leucine enkephalin, and have downregulated mu opioid receptors *(41–44)*. A multitude of endogenous pruritogens have now been identified, including acetylcholine, endothelins, kallilkreins, proteases, leukotrienes, prostaglandins, and more. What role each of these might have in cholestatic pruritus is still unexplored.

2.3. Therapy

First-line therapy in the treatment of cholestatic pruritus is bile acid binding resins, such as cholestyramine, because of their proven efficacy and safety (Table 2). According to a placebo-controlled trial, 80–85% of patients completely or partially respond to cholestyramine within 4–11 d, with relief being maintained for up to 32 mo *(45)*. The typical dose is 4–16 g/d in divided doses. Treatment with this agent is limited by its interference with absorption of other drugs and gastrointestinal side effects, such as constipation.

Rifampin is another efficacious agent in the treatment of pruritus *(46–48)*. It induces the P450 system and inhibits the hepatic transport of bile acids *(49,50)*. Phenobarbital, an equally potent inducer of the P450 system, does not decrease pruritus as much as rifampin; suggesting that the observed clinical effect of rifampin may not be entirely because of induction of the P450 system *(51)*. Rifampin has also been shown to be both safe and effective in children with cholestatic disease, with a greater effect in those with intrahepatic cholestasis compared to those with extrahepatic causes *(52)*. The typical dose in adults is 300–600 mg/d in divided doses and 10 mg/kg/d in children. A few case reports have described severe hepatotoxicity in some patients treated with rifampin *(53)*.

Based on experimental evidence that opioids are important mediators of itch, opioid antagonists have been studied in the treatment of cholestatic pruritus. Nalmefene, an oral opioid antagonist, improves pruritus as well as plasma bile acid concentrations in patients with cholestatic liver disease. The starting dose is usually 4–10 mg/d, which is then gradually titrated up every 2 d to achieve symptomatic control; the maximum studied dose is 240 mg/d *(54,55)*. A double-blinded, randomized controlled crossover trial of 29 cholestatic patients given naloxone (4 mg intravenous bolus, followed by 0.2 µg/kg/min) showed significant improvement in pruritus over 4 d *(56)*. Another double-blinded, randomized control trial of naltrexone (50 mg/d orally) in 16 cholestatic patients showed a significant improvement in pruritus within 4 wk *(57)*. Varying degrees of severity of a withdrawal-like reaction, characterized by anorexia, nausea, colicky abdominal pain, pallor, cool skin, and increased blood pressure have been reported in cholestatic patients treated with opioid antagonists. The reaction may begin within hours of administration, but the effect is temporary and usually subsides within 2–3 d, despite continued treatment. A breakthrough phenomenon, the sustained exacerbation of pruritus in the early weeks of treatment after an initial decrease, has been seen in 1 of 16 patients treated with naltrexone and 5 of 14 patients treated with nalmefene *(54,57)*. This effect may be because of the reversal of the downregulated opiate receptors in the brain during therapy. Unmasking of chronic pain can also occur with prolonged treatment *(58)*.

Serotonin is a newly recognized important neurotransmitter in the perception of pruritus. Sertraline, a selective serotonin reuptake inhibitor, was associated with improvement in cholestatic pruritus in one retrospective study *(59)*. A recent pilot study of sertraline (75–100 mg/d) demonstrated a significant improvement in visual analog scores, scratching activity, duration, and distribution of itch in those treated with sertraline as compared to placebo *(60)*. Initial studies of ondansetron, a 5-HT-3 antagonist, showed a small, but significant positive effect on pruritus *(61)*, but a subsequent double-blinded, randomized control trial showed that there was no difference in effect *(62)*. The mechanism by which serotonin modulates the perception of itch is still not known. Further studies are needed to evaluate the role and efficacy of serotonergic agents in the treatment of pruritus before they can be routinely recommended.

Other proposed therapies include grapefruit juice, dronabinol, plasmapheresis, and molecular adsorbent recirculating system (MARS). Small studies of PBC patients treated with 600 cc of daily grapefruit juice show some improvement in pruritic symptoms *(63)*. However, subsequent studies have been unable to produce similar results *(64)*. Patients with refractory pruritus treated with plasmapheresis had prompt relief of their symptoms, but the duration of this effect was variable from 1 d to 5 mo *(65)*. Patients with liver failure and cholestasis treated with MARS show an associated improvement in hepatic function and disappearance of pruritus *(66)*. The duration of effect is highly variable lasting from a few days to several months, even disappearing completely in several case reports and series *(67–69)*. A small case series of patients treated with dronabinol showed a brief antipruritic effect, lasting approximately 4–6 h *(70)*. Ursodeoxycholic acid (UDCA) and prednisone are associated with little to no relief in pruritus *(71)* of chronic cholestatic liver diseases, even though UDCA is quite effective in cholestasis of pregnancy.

3. DYSLIPIDEMIA

3.1. Prevalence

Patients with chronic cholestasis often have abnormalities in their lipid profiles. At the time of the first visit, approximately 75% of PBC patients have total cholesterol above 200 mg/dl. A cross-sectional study in patients with PBC showed that patients with early and intermediate histologic stages have mild elevations of very low density lipoproteins and low-density lipoproteins (LDLs) and marked increases in high-density lipoproteins (HDLs). In contrast, patients with advanced disease had marked elevations in LDLs with the presence of lipoprotein-X and a significant decrease in HDL *(72)*. The implications of this finding with respect to coronary artery disease, cerebrovascular disease, and overall morbidity and mortality are poorly understood. Despite marked hypercholesterolemia, excess mortality from cardiovascular disease has not been associated with PBC *(73)*. A prospective observational study of 312 PBC patients followed for 7.4 yr showed no statistical difference in the incidence of atherosclerotic death when compared to age- and sex-matched controls *(74)*.

3.2. Pathophysiology

The reason for the observed lack of cardiovascular events in patients with cholestatic dyslipidemia may be related to the difference in composition of the LDLs. Cholestatic patients have elevated levels of lipoprotein-X, which may be protective against atherogenesis *(75)*. However, lipoprotein-X may also contribute to hypercholesterolemia in cholestatic patients by not effectively downregulating hepatic hydroxymethylglutaryl coenzyme A reductase *(76)*.

3.3. Therapy

A small study of six PBC patients treated with simvastatin, a 3-hydroxy-3-methylglutaryl coenzyme A reductase inhibitor, showed a significant reduction in total cholesterol, LDL cholesterol, alkaline phosphatase, γ-glutamyltransferase, and immunoglobulin M *(77)*. Pravastatin, another HMG-coA reductase inhibitor, at 20 mg/d showed marked decrease in cholesterol and total bile acid levels, with pronounced decreases in cholic acid and chenodeoxycholic acid *(78)*. The use of reductase inhibitors is increasing in patients with cholestatic liver disease without subsequent reports of hepatotoxicity. However, further studies regarding clinical benefit and risk are needed before HMG-coA reductase inhibitors can be routinely recommended in cholestatic patients.

4. VITAMIN DEFICIENCY

4.1. Prevalence

Patients with cholestatic liver disease rarely present with symptoms of vitamin deficiencies. However, in a randomized, placebo-controlled trial evaluating the efficacy of UDCA in 180 patients with PBC at the Mayo Clinic, the proportion of patients with vitamin A, D, E, and K deficiency was 33.5%, 13.2%, 1.9%, and 7.8%, respectively *(79)*. Significant underlying disease, represented by advanced histologic stages, elevated Mayo risk score, and low cholesterol levels in a multivariate analysis, is associated with vitamin A deficiency. A Mayo risk score of 5 or greater has the highest sensitivity and specificity in identifying patients at risk for vitamin A deficiency. Similarly, low vitamin D levels are associated with low serum albumin *(79)*. Data regarding the prevalence of vitamin E deficiency are conflicting. One study comprising 42 patients with PBC found 43.5% to have vitamin E deficiency, all of whom exhibited clinically evident neurologic abnormalities manifested by poor scores on neuropsychologic testing measuring psychomotor capacity *(80)*. Another study evaluating the vitamin E status of patients with chronic liver disease showed 44% of PBC patients and 32% of patients with other cholestatic conditions to be deficient in vitamin E. Five of the 12 patients with both PBC and vitamin E deficiency demonstrated a mixed sensorimotor peripheral neuropathy, not characteristic of vitamin E deficiency *(81)*. Interestingly, this study demonstrated that those with very low levels of vitamin E were not readily corrected with oral, or even parenteral repletion, but those with less severe deficiencies were.

Table 3
Treatment Options for Vitamin Deficiency

Vitamin	Replacement	Maintenance
Vitamin A	50,000 IU/d	10,000 IU/d
Vitamin D	1600 IU/d	400 IU/d
Vitamin E	10 IU/kg/d	30 IU/d
Vitamin K	50 mg/d	5 mg/d

4.2. Pathophysiology

Patients with cholestatic liver disease are at risk for fat-soluble vitamin deficiencies because of the decreased availability of bile salts required for their absorption. Vitamin deficiencies usually occur well before overt symptoms of fat malabsorption. Poor absorption may be exacerbated by bile acid binding resins given for pruritus.

4.3. Therapy

Patients with early stage disease should be advised to consume a diet or multivitamin containing at least the RDA for the fat-soluble vitamins (700 mcg vitamin A, 10 mcg vitamin D, 16,000 mcg vitamin E, and 90 mcg vitamin K). Patients with advanced cholestatic liver disease at risk for fat-soluble vitamin deficiencies should be tested annually to identify deficiencies and treated with replacement doses followed by maintenance therapy (Table 3). Of note, serum for vitamin A levels must be drawn into a light-proof vial, and vitamin E levels may be falsely elevated in patients with hyperlipidemia. A serum vitamin E to total lipid ratio of <0.8 mcg/g is considered deficient.

5. SUMMARY

Though cholestasis is a common clinical problem, it is important to understand that recommendations regarding the management of complications of cholestasis are based on trials consisting of small numbers of patients, predominantly with PBC, and are thus based largely on clinical experience. Osteoporosis is very common in patients with cholestatic liver disease when compared to the general population. Treatment goals are to prevent further bone loss, thereby reducing the risk of fracture. Bisphosphonates, hormone replacement therapy, and vitamin K all increase BMD and prevent further bone loss in cholestatic patients. Management of pruritus resulting from cholestasis remains challenging because of incomplete understanding of the mechanisms involved and the limited array of effective therapies. Current treatment is aimed at reducing bile acid concentration, reducing opioid tonicity, modulating serotonergic activity, and dialysis of as yet unidentified pruritogens. Though patients with cholestatic liver disease exhibit dyslipidemia and these levels can be reduced with the use of HMG-coA reductase inhibitors, the long-term impact of therapy on vascular events remains controversial and provides opportunity for further clinical investigation. Finally, patients with advanced cholestatic liver disease are at risk for vitamin deficiencies, particularly vitamins A and D, and thus should be screened and treated when found to be deficient.

REFERENCES

1. Sokhi RP, Anantharaju A, Kondaveeti R, Creech SD, Islam KK, and Van Thiel DH. Bone mineral density among cirrhotic patients awaiting liver transplantation. Liver Transplant 2004; 10(5): 648–653.
2. Menon KV, Angulo P, Weston S, Dickson ER, and Lindor KD. Bone disease in PBC: independent indicators and rate of progression. J Hepatol 2001; 35(3): 316–323.
3. Hay JE, Lindor KD, Wiesner RH, Dickson ER, Krom RA, and LaRusso NF. The metabolic bone disease of primary sclerosing cholangitis. Hepatology 1991; 14(2): 257–261.
4. Guichelaar MM, Malinchoc M, Sibonga JD, Clarke BL, and Hay JE. Bone histomorphometric changes after liver transplantation for chronic cholestatic liver disease. J Bone Miner Res 2003; 18(12): 2190–2199.
5. Argao EA, Specker BL, and Heubi JE. Bone mineral content in infants and children with chronic cholestatic liver disease. Pediatrics 1993; 91(6): 1151–1154.
6. Xu H and Eichstaedt H. Assessment of serial changes of bone mineral density at lumbar spine and femoral neck before and after liver transplantation. Chin Med J (Engl.) 1999; 112(4): 379–381.
7. Hay JE and Guichelaar MM. Evaluation and management of osteoporosis in liver disease. Clin Liver Dis 2005; 9(4): 747–766.
8. Guanabens N, Pares A, Ros I, et al. Severity of cholestasis and advanced histological stage but not menopausal status are the major risk factors for osteoporosis in PBC. J Hepatol 2005; 42(4): 573–577.
9. Guichelaar MM, Malinchoc M, Sibonga J, Clarke BL, and Hay JE. Bone metabolism in advanced cholestatic liver disease: analysis by bone histomorphometry. Hepatology 2002; 36(4 Pt 1): 895–903.
10. Skinner RK, Sherlock S, Long RG, and Wilis MR. 25-Hydroxylation of vitamin D in PBC. Lancet 1977; 1(8014): 720–721.
11. Kaplan MM, Goldberg MJ, Matloff DS, Neer RM, and Goodman DB. Effect of 25-hydroxyvitamin D3 on vitamin D metabolites in PBC. Gastroenterology 1981; 81(4): 681–685.
12. Matloff DS, Kaplan MM, Neer RM, Goldberg MJ, Bitman W, and Wolfe HJ. Osteoporosis in PBC: effects of 25-hydroxyvitamin D3 treatment. Gastroenterology 1982; 83(1 Pt 1): 97–102.
13. Herlong HF, Recker RR, and Maddrey WC. Bone disease in PBC: histologic features and response to 25-hydroxyvitamin D. Gastroenterology 1982; 83(1 Pt 1): 103–108.

14. Crippin JS, Jorgensen RA, Dickson ER, and Lindor KD. Hepatic osteodystrophy in PBC: effects of medical treatment. Am J Gastroenterol 1994; 89(1): 47–50.

15. Pares A, Guanabens N, and Rodes J. Gene polymorphisms as predictors of decreased bone mineral density and osteoporosis in PBC. Eur J Gastroenterol Hepatol 2005; 17(3): 311–315.

16. Lakatos LP, Bajnok E, Hegedus D, Toth T, Lakatos P, and Szalay F. Vitamin D receptor, oestrogen receptor-alpha gene and interleukin-1 receptor antagonist gene polymorphisms in Hungarian patients with PBC. Eur J Gastroenterol Hepatol 2002; 14(7): 733–740.

17. Koshihara Y, Hoshi K, Ishibashi H, and Shiraki M. Vitamin K2 promotes 1alpha, 25(OH)2 vitamin D3-induced mineralization in human periosteal osteoblasts. Calcif. Tissue Int 1996; 59(6): 466–473.

18. Kameda T, Miyazawa K, Mori Y, et al. Vitamin K2 inhibits osteoclastic bone resorption by inducing osteoclast apoptosis Biochem Biophys. Res Commun 1996; 220(3): 515–519.

19. Iwamoto J, Takeda T, and Sato Y. Effects of vitamin K2 on osteoporosis. Curr Pharm Des 2004; 10(21): 2557–2576.

20. Shiomi S, Nishiguchi S, Kubo S, et al. Vitamin K2 (menatetrenone) for bone loss in patients with cirrhosis of the liver. Am J Gastroenterol 2002; 97(4): 978–981.

21. Janes CH, Dickson ER, Okazaki R, Bonde S, McDonagh AF, and Riggs BL. Role of hyperbilirubinemia in the impairment of osteoblast proliferation associated with cholestatic jaundice. J Clin Invest 1995; 95(6): 2581–2586.

22. Olsson R, Mattsson LA, Obrant K, and Mellstrom D. Estrogen–progestogen therapy for low bone mineral density in PBC. Liver 1999; 19(3): 188–192.

23. Menon KV, Angulo P, Boe GM, and Lindor KD. Safety and efficacy of estrogen therapy in preventing bone loss in PBC. Am J Gastroenterol 2003; 98(4): 889–892.

24. Ettinger B, Black DM, Mitlak BH, et al. Reduction of vertebral fracture risk in postmenopausal women with osteoporosis treated with raloxifene: results from a 3-year randomized clinical trial. Multiple Outcomes of Raloxifene Evaluation (MORE) Investigators. JAMA 1999; 282(7): 637–645.

25. Levy C, Harnois DM, Angulo P, Jorgensen R, and Lindor KD. Raloxifene improves bone mass in osteopenic women with PBC: results of a pilot study. Liver Int 2005; 25(1): 117–121.

26. Guanabens N, Pares A, del Rio L, et al. Sodium fluoride prevents bone loss in PBC. J Hepatol 1992; 15(3): 345–349.

27. Guanabens N, Pares A, Monegal A, et al. Etidronate versus fluoride for treatment of osteopenia in PBC: preliminary results after 2 years. Gastroenterology 1997; 113(1): 219–224.

28. Lindor KD, Jorgensen RA, Tiegs RD, Khosla S, and Dickson ER. Etidronate for osteoporosis in primary biliary cirrhosis: a randomized trial. J Hepatol 2000; 33(6): 878–882.

29. Guanabens N, Pares A, Ros I, et al. Alendronate is more effective than etidronate for increasing bone mass in osteopenic patients with PBC. Am J Gastroenterol 2003; 98(10): 2268–2274.

30. Zein CO, Jorgensen RA, Clarke B, et al. Alendronate improves bone mineral density in primary biliary cirrhosis: a randomized placebo-controlled trial. Hepatology 2005; (4): 1 762–771.

31. Camisasca M, Crosignani A, Battezzati PM, et al. Parenteral calcitonin for metabolic bone disease associated with PBC. Hepatology 1994; 20(3): 633–637.

32. Hay JE, Malinchoc M, and Dickson ER. A controlled trial of calcitonin therapy for the prevention of post-liver transplantation atraumatic fractures in patients with PBC and primary sclerosing cholangitis. J Hepatol 2001; 34(2): 292–298.
33. Potts JT. Parathyroid hormone: past and present. J Endocrinol 2005; 187(3): 311–325.
34. Adams J and Pepping J. Vitamin K in the treatment and prevention of osteoporosis and arterial calcification. Am J Health Syst Pharm 2005; 62(15): 1574–1581.
35. Nishiguchi S, Shimoi S, Kurooka H, et al. Randomized pilot trial of vitamin K2 for bone loss in patients with PBC. J Hepatol 2001; 35(4): 543–545.
36. Mela M, Mancuso A, and Burroughs AK. Review article: pruritus in cholestatic and other liver diseases. Aliment Pharmacol Ther 2003; 17(7): 857–870.
37. Varadi DP. Pruritus induced by crude bile and purified bile acids. Experimental production of pruritus in human skin. Arch Dermatol 1974; 109(5): 678–681.
38. O'Keeffe C, Baird AW, Nolan N, and McCormick PA. Cholestatic pruritus—the role of cutaneous mast cells and nerves. Aliment Pharmacol Ther 2004; 19(12): 1293–1300.
39. Jones EA and Zylicz Z. Treatment of pruritus caused by cholestasis with opioid antagonists. J Palliat Med 2005; 8(6): 1290–1294.
40. Koenigstein H. Experimental study of itch stimuli in animals. Arch Dermatol Syph 1948; 57: 828–849.
41. Swain MG, Rothman RB, Xu H, Vergalla J, Bergasa NV, and Jones EA. Endogenous opioids accumulate in plasma in a rat model of acute cholestasis. Gastroenterology 1992; 103(2): 630–635.
42. Nelson L, Vergnolle N, D'Mello C, Chapman K, Le T, and Swain MG. Endogenous opioid-mediated antinociception in cholestatic mice is peripherally, not centrally, mediated. J Hepatol 2005; 27: 1–9.
43. Kuraishi Y, Yamaguchi T, and Miyamoto T. Itch-scratch responses induced by opioids through central mu opioid receptors in mice. J Biomed Sci 2000; 7(3): 248–252.
44. Bergasa NV, Rothman RB, Vergalla J, Xu H, Swain MG, and Jones EA. Central mu-opioid receptors are down-regulated in a rat model of cholestasis. J Hepatol 1991; 15(1–2): 220–224.
45. Datta DV and Sherlock S. Cholestyramine for long term relief of the pruritus complicating Intrahepatic cholestasis. Gastroenterology 1966; 50(3): 323–332.
46. Price TJ, Patterson WK, and Olver IN. Rifampicin as treatment for pruritus in malignant cholestasis. Support Care Cancer 1998; 6(6): 533–535.
47. Bachs L, Pares A, Elena M, Piera C, and Rodes J. Effects of long-term rifampicin administration in PBC. Gastroenterology 1992; 102(6): 2077–2080.
48. Podesta A, Lopez P, Terg R, et al. Treatment of pruritus of PBC with rifampin. Dig Dis Sci 1991; 36(2): 216–220.
49. Miguet JP, Mavier P, Soussy CJ, and Dhumeaux D. Induction of hepatic microsomal enzymes after brief administration of rifampicin in man. Gastroenterology 1977; 72(5 Pt 1): 924–926.
50. Galeazzi R, Lorenzini I, and Orlandi F. Rifampicin-induced elevation of serum bile acids in man. Dig Dis Sci 1980; 25(2): 108–112.
51. Bachs L, Pares A, Elena M, Piera C, and Rodes J. Comparison of rifampicin with phenobarbitone for treatment of pruritus in biliary cirrhosis. Lancet 1989; 1(8638): 574–576.
52. Yerushalmi B, Sokol RJ, Narkewicz MR, Smith D, and Karrer FM. Use of rifampin for severe pruritus in children with chronic cholestasis. J Pediatr Gastroenterol Nutr 1999; 29(4): 442–447.

53. Prince MI, Burt AD, and Jones DE. Hepatitis and liver dysfunction with rifampicin therapy for pruritus in primary biliary cirrhosis. Gut 2002; 50(3): 436–439.

54. Bergasa NV, Alling DW, Talbot TL, Wells MC, and Jones EA. Oral nalmefene therapy reduces scratching activity due to the pruritus of cholestasis: a controlled study. J Am Acad Dermatol 1999; 41(3 Pt 1): 431–434.

55. Thornton JR and Losowsky MS. Opioid peptides and PBC. BMJ 1988; 297(6662): 1501–1504.

56. Bergasa NV, Alling DW, Talbot TL, et al. Effects of naloxone infusions in patients with the pruritus of cholestasis. A double-blind, randomized, controlled trial. Ann Intern Med 1995; 123(3): 161–167.

57. Wolfhagen FH, Sternieri E, Hop WC, Vitale G, Bertolotti M, and Van Buuren HR. Oral naltrexone treatment for cholestatic pruritus: a double-blind, placebo-controlled study. Gastroenterology 1997; 113(4): 1264–1269.

58. McRae CA, Prince MI, Hudson M, Day CP, James O, and Jones D. Pain as a complication of use of opiate antagonists for symptom control in cholestasis. Gastroenterology 2003; 125(2): 591–596.

59. Browning J, Combes B, and Mayo MJ. Long-term efficacy of sertraline as a treatment for cholestatic pruritus in patients with PBC. Am J Gastroenterol 2003; 98(12): 2736–2741.

60. Mayo M, Handem I, Saldana S, Jacobe H, Getachew Y, and Rush AJ. Effect of sertraline on pruritus in cholestatic liver disease: a randomized double blind placebo controlled crossover study. Hepatology 2005; 42(4 Suppl 1): 209A.

61. Muller C, Pongratz S, Pidlich J, et al. Treatment of pruritus in chronic liver disease with the 5-hydroxytryptamine receptor type 3 antagonist ondansetron: a randomized, placebo-controlled, double-blind cross-over trial. Eur J Gastroenterol Hepatol 1998; 10(10): 865–870.

62. O'Donohue JW, Pereira SP, Ashdown AC, Haigh CG, Wilkinson JR, and Williams R. A controlled trial of ondansetron in the pruritus of cholestasis. Aliment Pharmacol Ther 2005; 21(8): 1041–1045.

63. Horsmans Y and Geubel AP. Pruritus associated with cholestatic liver disease. Ann Intern Med 1996; 125(8): 701.

64. Cadranel JF, Di Martino V, and Devergie B. Grapefruit juice for the pruritus of cholestatic liver disease. Ann Intern Med 1997; 126(11): 920–921.

65. Lauterburg BH, Taswell HF, Pineda AA, Dickson ER, Burgstaler EA, and Carlson GL. Treatment of pruritus of cholestasis by plasma perfusion through USP-charcoal-coated glass beads. Lancet 1980; 2(8185): 53–55.

66. Stange J, Hassanein TI, Mehta R, Mitzner SR, and Bartlett RH. The molecular adsorbents recycling system as a liver support system based on albumin dialysis: a summary of preclinical investigations, prospective, randomized, controlled clinical trial, and clinical experience from 19 centers. Artif. Organs 2002; 26(2): 103–110.

67. Acevedo Ribo M, Moreno Planas JM, Sanz Moreno C, et al. Therapy of intractable pruritus with MARS. Transplant Proc 2005; 37(3): 1480–1481.

68. Bellmann R, Graziadei IW, Feistritzer C, et al. Treatment of refractory cholestatic pruritus after liver transplantation with albumin dialysis. Liver Transplant 2004; 10(1): 107–114.

69. Pares A, Cisneros L, Salmeron JM, et al. Extracorporeal albumin dialysis: a procedure for prolonged relief of intractable pruritus in patients with PBC. Am J Gastroenterol 2004; 99(6): 1105–1110.

70. Neff GW, O'Brien CB, Reddy KR, et al. Preliminary observation with dronabinol in patients with intractable pruritus secondary to cholestatic liver disease. Am J Gastroenterol 2002; 97(8): 2117–2119.
71. Gluud C and Christensen E. Ursodeoxycholic acid for PBC. Cochrane Database Syst Rev 2002; (1): CD000551.
72. Jahn CE, Schaefer EJ, Taam LA, et al. Lipoprotein abnormalities in PBC. Association with hepatic lipase inhibition as well as altered cholesterol esterification. Gastroenterology 1985; 89(6): 1266–1278.
73. Longo M, Crosignani A, Battezzati PM, et al. Hyperlipidaemic state and cardiovascular risk in PBC. Gut 2002; 51(2): 265–269.
74. Crippin JS, Lindor KD, Jorgensen R, et al. Hypercholesterolemia and atherosclerosis in PBC: what is the risk? Hepatology 1992; 15(5): 858–862.
75. Agorastos J, Fox C, Harry DS, and McIntyre N. Lecithin–cholesterol acyltransferase and the lipoprotein abnormalities of obstructive jaundice. Clin Sci Mol Med 1978; 54(4): 369–379.
76. Edwards CM, Otal MP, and Stacpoole PW. Lipoprotein-X fails to inhibit hydroxymethylglutaryl coenzyme A reductase in HepG2 cells. Metabolism 1993; 42(7): 807–813.
77. Ritzel U, Leonhardt U, Nather M, Schafer G, Armstrong VW, and Ramadori G. Simvastatin in PBC: effects on serum lipids and distinct disease markers. J Hepatol 2002; 36(4): 454–458.
78. Kurihara T, Akimoto M, Abe K, et al. Experimental use of pravastatin in patients with PBC associated with hypercholesterolemia. Clin Ther 1993; 15(5): 890–898.
79. Phillips JR, Angulo P, Petterson T, and Lindor KD. Fat-soluble vitamin levels in patients with PBC. Am J Gastroenterol 2001; 96(9): 2745–2750.
80. Arria AM, Tarter RE, Warty V, and Van Thiel DH. Vitamin E deficiency and psychomotor dysfunction in adults with PBC. Am J Clin Nutr 1990; 52(2): 383–390.
81. Jeffrey GP, Muller DP, Burroughs AK, et al. Vitamin E deficiency and its clinical significance in adults with PBC and other forms of chronic liver disease. J Hepatol 1987; 4(3): 307–317.

10 Cholestasis Post Liver Transplantation

Kymberly D. S. Watt and Timothy M. McCashland

CONTENTS

Abstract

Cholestasis occurs frequently after liver transplantation and has a very broad differential diagnosis. Cholestasis can occur anytime throughout the posttransplant period and may be intrahepatic or extrahepatic in origin. This chapter reviews the common causes of cholestasis in the posttransplant setting.

Key Words: Cholestasis; liver transplant; biliary complications.

Cholestasis is common after a liver transplant and occurs when the process of bile production or bile flow is impeded. This can happen within the extrahepatic biliary system or at the intrahepatic or cellular

From: *Clinical Gastroenterology: Cholestatic Liver Disease*
Edited by: K. D. Lindor and J. A. Talwalkar © Humana Press Inc., Totowa, NJ

Table 1
Causes of Cholestasis After Liver Transplantation

Early (<6 mo)	*Late (>6 mo)*
Extrahepatic:	**Extrahepatic:**
Stricture—single (anastomotic, external compression)	Benign Stricture—Single (anastomotic)
Stricture—multiple (HAT/ischemic)	Multiple (HAT/ischemic, rPSC)
Biliary leak	Malignant stricture—cholangiocarcinoma
Cholangitis	Stones
Intrahepatic:	**Intrahepatic:**
Preservation/reperfusion injury	Acute cellular rejection
ABO incompatibility	Chronic rejection
HAT	Drug induced
Small for size graft	Recurrent disease (PBC, PSC, viral)
Drug induced	*Denovo* viral hepatitis, autoimmune disease
Acute cellular rejection	
Sepsis	
Infection—CMV, bacterial, fungal, FCH	

HAT, hepatic artery thrombosis; rPSC, recurrent primary sclerosing cholangitis; CMV, cytomegalovirus infection; FCH, fibrosing cholestatic hepatitis; PBC, primary biliary cirrhosis; PSC, primary sclerosing cholangitis.

level. Depending on the underlying reason for the cholestasis, the short- and long-term consequences can range from minimal to severe.

The differential diagnosis of cholestasis post liver transplantation is broad. It is commonly interpreted in terms of early cholestatic syndromes (<6 mo) and late cholestatic syndromes (>6 mo) relative to the operative procedure, but considerable overlap can occur. Within these timeframes, both intrahepatic and extrahepatic causes exist. Table 1 outlines these concepts.

1. BILIARY COMPLICATIONS

Biliary complications in the early postoperative setting include biliary leaks and biliary obstruction related to both anastomotic and nonana-stomotic strictures, with secondary cholangitis as a possible consequence. Biliary complications occur in 10–50% of transplants with associated mortality rates of 0–20%, anastomosis revision rates of 12–25%, and retransplantation rates of 6–12% *(1–4)*. The benefit and use of T-tubes in reducing these complications is still debated *(2–4)*. Higher rates of biliary complications after a Roux-en-Y anastomosis is thought to be representative of its use in more complicated procedures (i.e., retransplantation and diffuse extrahepatic disease such as primary sclerosing cholangitis [PSC]) *(3)*.

The majority of biliary leaks will resolve with nonoperative intervention, whereas anastomotic biliary strictures are more likely to require surgical correction. Endoscopic and percutaneous biliary stenting is frequently the first intervention for these strictures with the highest success rates (60–75%) with biliary stents and dilatation compared to dilatation alone *(5)*. These procedures are more successful in early strictures (<6 mo) as compared to late strictures (>6 mo) *(3)*.

Nonanastomotic strictures occur at a frequency of 2–20% *(6)*. They tend be multifocal, can be both intrahepatic and extrahepatic, and are more likely to require surgical intervention including retransplantation. They can occur early (<6 mo) or late (>6 mo) and are associated with several underlying causes including hepatic artery thrombosis (HAT), warm and cold/ischemic injury, ABO incompatibility, recurrent PSC, and possibly viral infections such as cytomegalovirus (CMV) or even hepatitis C (HCV), which are discussed in more detail in later sections *(6,7)*. Graft survival appears to be significantly lower in patients with nonanastomotic strictures compared to matched patients without stricturing *(6)*.

Impacted biliary stones generally occur later post transplant and are often associated with biliary strictures and impaired bile flow and respond to endoscopic treatment *(1)*. Medications including cyclosporine may increase the risk of stone formation in the transplant setting *(8)*.

2. PRESERVATION/REPERFUSION INJURY AND ABO INCOMPATIBILITY

Preservation injury has been reported to occur in approximately 17% of transplants, but rates as high as 50% have been reported *(9,10)*. Extrahepatic biliary complications such as nonanastomotic strictures occur with increasing frequency as the cold ischemic time increases over 10–12 h *(9,10)*. Preservation injury also occurs at the cellular level, involving nonparenchymal cells (sinusoidal endothelial cell injury and Kupffer cell activation, with accumulation of inflammatory cells and platelets) as well as parenchymal cells including biliary epithelial cells *(11,12)*. Histological findings of preservation/reperfusion injury include neutrophilic infiltration, microvesicular steatosis, hepatocyte cytoaggregation that occurs early and progresses to centrilobular necrosis, hepatocyte swelling, and cholestasis later in the process *(10)*. Mild cases resolve spontaneously, but more severe cases may have residual damage or result in primary nonfunction *(10)*. Expansion of the donor pool with donation after cardiac death and the biliary complications with these allografts are thought to be because of prolonged warm ischemic time *(13)*.

Blood group related antigens (ABO) are expressed on the epithelial cells of large bile ducts and periductular hepatocytes *(14)*. Thus, the hepatic allograft may be more susceptible to immunologic bile duct injury after transplantation across the ABO barrier. Complication rates such as biliary structuring, HAT, and cellular rejection were significantly higher in these patients *(7)*. Graft survival and patient survival have been inferior to ABO matched transplants in retrospective studies *(7)*. Blood group O recipients appear to have better outcomes compared to blood group A and B recipients.

3. SMALL FOR SIZE SYNDROME

Small for size syndrome (SFSS) is a recognized complication when the recipient receives inadequate functional tissue and is thought to occur at a graft to recipient body weight ratio less than 0.8. The presentation can vary from mild isolated hyperbilirubinemia to graft failure. Within the first week of transplant the patient may develop cholestasis, prolonged coagulation, ascites, and variceal bleeding *(15)*. Histologic examination shows bilirubin plugs and cholestasis with patchy areas of necrosis and regenerative tissue *(15)*. The physiologic mechanisms of SFSS are not clear but suspected to be related to portal hyperperfusion and arterial hypoperfusion resulting in endothelial disruption and subsequent molecular derangements on the hepatic regeneration process *(15)*.

4. HEPATIC ARTERY THROMBOSIS

HAT is described in 3–9% of transplants, with another 3% of patients experiencing nonthrombotic complications such as hepatic artery stenosis, redundancy, and pseudoaneurysm *(16)*. In the transplanted liver, HAT results in more significant biliary damage compared to a nontransplanted liver because of the surgical excision interrupting smaller peripheral arteries that would normally supply collateral flow *(16)*. One-third of HAT occurs within the first month and may present with cholestasis *(17)*. As the main blood supply to the biliary system stems from the hepatic artery, later complications tend to include bile duct stricturing with subsequent cholangitis, liver abscess, biloma, and/or biliary necrosis with bile leak. Either the early or late presentation can progress to severe liver failure *(17,18)*. Retransplantation rates of 50–80% and mortality rates of up to 50–70% have been described in patients with HAT *(17–19)*.

Risk factors for HAT include not only vascular surgical technique but also biliary anastomosis (Roux-en-Y), bile leaks, cold and warm ischemic injury, antibody cross-match status, coagulation abnormalities, infections (particularly CMV), and possible immunologic factors *(18,19)*. An increased risk has been associated with cigarette smoking in both the pretransplant setting and the posttransplant setting *(20)*. Interventional radiology procedures (such as angioplasty and fibrinolysis) or immediate surgical revascularization are needed to avoid retransplantation *(18,21)*.

5. INFECTIOUS COMPLICATIONS

5.1. Bacterial and Fungal

Cholestasis with or without hyperbilirubinemia is frequently associated with extrahepatic bacterial or fungal infections and sepsis *(22)*. Evidence suggests that proinflammatory cytokines and endotoxin release are potent inhibitors of hepatobiliary transporter gene expression resulting in hyperbilirubinemia and cholestasis *(23)*. Although seldom necessary, histological assessment may reveal nonspecific cholestasis and hepatitis or a neutrophilic infiltration of the bile ducts, biliary proliferation, and bile plugs termed 'cholangitis lenta' *(24)*.

5.2. Viral

CMV is a common viral pathogen in liver transplant recipients and is reported in 30–80% of transplant patients with up to 30% of patients developing CMV disease and 12–17% CMV hepatitis. The highest risk is within the first 3–4 mo post transplant *(22,25)*. CMV can infect and injure not only hepatocytes, but also biliary epithelium and vascular endothelium *(26,27)* and thus can present as cholestasis. Histologic findings can range from lymphocytic infiltration, ballooned hepatocytes, cholangitis, cholestasis, endothelitis, and Kupffer cell reaction to more specific findings of microabcesses or rarely viral inclusions *(28)*. CMV has been implicated in vanishing bile duct syndrome and both acute and chronic rejection *(26–28)*.

Human herpesvirus-6 and -7 (HHV-6 and -7) activations are common and usually associated with CMV infection and rejection in liver transplant patients *(29)*. They may present with cholestasis in a similar manner that CMV presents. Herpes simplex virus (HSV) as well as toxoplasmosis should also be considered in the immunosuppressed patient in appropriate settings *(22)*. Hepatitis C and hepatitis B viral (HBV) infections are discussed below.

6. DRUG INDUCED

Drugs and toxins are a common cause of cholestasis and can be the result of direct injury to the cells or via an idiosyncratic reaction to the drug. Many of the commonly used drugs including immuno-suppressive drugs, antibiotics, antifungals, and antivirals should be considered in the workup of cholestasis. We will only review the immunosuppressive medications.

Cyclosporine induces cholestasis by decreasing both bile flow and bile salt secretion. Its suppression of bile salt synthesis reduces the bile salt pool size *(30)*. The drug inhibits bile salt and phospholipid secretion without a corresponding change in cholesterol secretion and thus elevates cholesterol saturation in bile, a potential risk for gallstone formation *(8,30)*. In contrast, tacrolimus has been shown to have higher bile flow rates and more rapid recovery of bile flow post transplantation compared to cyclosporine *(31)*. However, cholestasis also been attributed to tacrolimus which may be because of deranged bile acid transport or related to impaired glutathione and bicarbonate excretion *(31,32)*. Sirolimus and everolimus also appear to have cholestatic effects by mechanisms resulting in retention of toxic metabolites within the hepatocytes *(32,33)*. Azathioprine can cause hepatotoxicity of a variety of mechanisms including cholestasis *(34)*.

7. ACUTE CELLULAR REJECTION AND CHRONIC REJECTION (CR)

The mechanism by which patients with acute cellular rejection (ACR) develop cholestasis is multifactorial and related to the lympho-cytic destruction of the small intrahepatic bile ducts or apoptosis of the biliary epithelial cell, and impaired bile secretion related to Kupffer cell-induced cytokine release *(35–37)*. If early acute cellular rejection is not treated or responds inadequately to treatment, then progression to irreversible injury and chronic rejection occurs.

Chronic 'ductopenic' rejection occurs in 2–5% of transplant patients and generally presents as cholestasis within 6 wk–12 mo of transplan-tation, but has been noted as early as 2- to 3-wk post-op *(38,39)*. It is characterized by progressive loss of intrahepatic interlobular and septal bile ducts (ductopenia) with lipid laden vasculopathy in 50% of portal tracts *(39)*. Risk factors for the development of CR include CMV infection, pretransplant disease etiology (PSC, primary biliary cirrhosis [PBC], and autoimmune hepatitis [AIH] have the highest incidence), HLA matching, donor male:recipient female status, number and severity of acute rejection episodes *(27,38)*. Whether the pathogenesis is related to an immune-mediated injury or an ischemic injury resulting from the obliterative arteritis is unclear *(16,40)*. Undoubtedly, the processes are linked and it is the combination and severity of each component that results in the clinical manifestation of chronic ductopenic rejection.

8. RECURRENT DISEASE

8.1. Primary Biliary Cirrhosis and Primary Sclerosing Cholangitis

PBC recurs in up to 17% of patients by 36 mo and 30–50% of patients by 10 yr *(41–43)*. Diagnosis is confirmed based on histologic findings of florid duct lesions or destructive lymphocytic cholangitis within a dense portal mononuclear inflammatory infiltrate, formation of lymphoid aggregates, and epithelioid granulomas *(41,42)*. Clear risk factors for recurrence have not been elucidated. The choice of immunosuppression was initially thought to be a risk factor, but recent studies do not demonstrate any significant influence on patient survival, PBC-related graft loss, or development of acute or chronic rejection episodes *(43)*.

Recurrent PSC is thought to occur in 9–20% of patients by 5 yr *(44–47)*. It is not a straightforward diagnosis as there is an increased incidence of both acute and chronic rejection, HAT, and biliary stricturing in these patients *(44–47)*. A combination of cholangiographic findings of intrahepatic and/or extrahepatic strictures and beading along with histologic findings including biliary fibrosis/cirrhosis, fibro-obliterative lesions, and cholangitis with or without ductopenia are required for the diagnosis *(44)*. Risk factors for recurrent disease have not been clearly delineated. Patients who received maintenance corticosteroids or orthoclone (OKT3) post transplant may be at higher risk of recurrent PSC *(47)*. Coexistent inflammatory bowel disease was associated with higher rates of recurrence but may be because of the steroid requirement *(47)*.

In PSC, risk of cholangiocarcinoma prior to transplant ranges from 7 to 13% over 10 yr but the risk in recurrent PSC is unknown *(48)*. Patients with known cholangiocarcinoma prior to transplant have extremely poor outcomes post transplant, and those with incidental tumors at transplant have a high risk of recurrent cholangiocarcinoma *(44,45,48)*. Overall survival rate for PSC patients with recurrent disease is similar to those without recurrence, but retransplantation is not uncommon *(48)*.

8.2. Viral Hepatitis

Recurrent viral hepatitis of any severity can present with cholestasis. Fibrosing cholestatic hepatitis (FCH) is a severe form of HBV and HCV recurrence or reactivation in the allograft that manifests clinically within weeks to months of transplantation as cholestasis and progresses rapidly to liver failure, if left untreated. The frequency of this entity in HBV-infected patients has decreased significantly since the introduction of prophylactic therapies to prevent HBV recurrence, but continues to occur in approximately 5–7% of patients transplanted for HCV *(49,50)*. It is thought to be a result of virus-specific cytopathic injury as opposed to immunologic injury. FCH is characterized histologically by periportal fibrosis, prominent cholestasis, and hepatocyte swelling progressing to centrilobular balloon degeneration and bridging fibrosis/cirrhosis *(49,50)*. Minimizing immunosuppression may reduce the risk of developing FCH, Early treatment with antiviral medications may delay the progression of disease and improve prognosis, but studies are lacking.

9. SUMMARY

Cholestasis is a frequent finding post liver transplantation with a very broad differential diagnosis. Timing of the cholestatic presentation may help to narrow the possibilities, but significant overlap exists. Careful diagnostic imaging of the biliary tree is an important first step in the workup, followed by liver biopsy if clinically indicated.

REFERENCES

1. Nemec P, Ondrasek J, Studenik P, Hokl J, and Cerny J. Biliary complications in liver transplantation. Ann Transplant 2001; 6(2): 24–28.
2. Kusano T, Randall HB, Roberts JP, and Ascher NL. The use of stents for duct-to-duct anastomoses of biliary reconstruction in orthotopic liver transplantation. Hepatogastroenterology 2005; 52(63): 695–699.
3. Thethy S, Thomson BNJ, Pleass H, et al. Management of biliary tract complications after orthotopic liver transplantation. Clin Transplant 2004; 18(6): 647–653.
4. Scatton O, Meunier B, Cherqui D, et al. Randomized trial of choledocho-choledochostomy with or without a T-tube in orthotopic liver transplantation. Ann Surg 2001; 233(3): 432–437.
5. Zoepf T, Maldonado-Lopez EJ, Hilgard P, et al. Balloon dilatation vs. balloon dilatation plus bile duct endoprostheses for treatment of anastomotic biliary strictures after liver transplantation. Liver Transplant 2006; 12(1): 88–94.
6. Guichelaar MM, Benson JT, Malinchoc M, et al. Risk factors for and clinical course of non-anastomotic biliary strictures after liver transplantation. Am J Transplant 2003; 3(7): 885–890.
7. Sanchez-Urdazpal L, Batts KP, Gores GJ, et al. Increased bile duct complications in liver transplantation across the ABO barrier. Ann Surg 1993; 218(2): 152–158.

8. Cadranel JF, Erlinger S, Desruenne M, et al. Chronic administration of cyclosporin A induces a decrease in hepatic excretory function in man. Dig Dis Sci 1992; 37(10): 1473–1476.

9. Busquets J, Figueras J, Serrano T, et al. Postreperfusion biopsies are useful in predicting complications after liver transplantation. Liver Transplant 2001; 7(5): 432–435.

10. Lee YM, Obrien CB, Yamashiki N, et al. Preservation injury patterns in liver transplantation associated with poor prognosis. Transpl Proc 2003; 35: 2964–2966.

11. Cutrin JC, Cantino D, Biasi F, et al. Reperfusion damage to the bile canaliculi in transplanted human liver. Hepatology 1996; 24(5): 1053–1057.

12. Kukan M, and Haddad PS. Role of hepatocytes and bile duct cells in preservation–reperfusion injury of liver grafts. Liver Transplant 2001; 7(5): 381–400.

13. Abt P, Crawford M, Desai N, et al. Liver transplantation from controlled non-heart-beating donors: an increased incidence of biliary complications. Transplantation 2003; 75(10): 1659–1663.

14. Nakanuma Y, and Sasaki M. Expression of blood group-related antigens in the intrahepatic biliary tree and hepatocytes in normal livers and various hepatobiliary diseases. Hepatology 1989; 10(2): 174–178.

15. Dahm F, Georgiev P, and Clavien PA. Small-for-size syndrome after partial liver transplantation: definition, mechanisms of disease and clinical implications. Am J Transplant 2005; 5(11): 2605–2610.

16. Deltenre P, and Valla DC. Ischemic cholangiopathy. J Hepatol 2006; 44: 806–817.

17. Jain A, Costa G, Marsh W, et al. Thrombotic and nonthrombotic hepatic artery complications in adults and children following primary liver transplantation with long-term follow-up in 1000 consecutive patients. Transplant Int 2006; 19(1): 27–37.

18. Silva MA, Jambulingam PS, Gunson BK, et al. Hepatic artery thrombosis following orthotopic liver transplantation: a 10-year experience from a single centre in the United Kingdom. Liver Transplant 2006; 12(1): 146–151.

19. Pastacaldi S, Teixeira R, Montalto P, Rolles K, and Burroughs AK. Hepatic artery thrombosis after orthotopic liver transplantation: a review of nonsurgical causes. Liver Transplant 2001; 7: 75–81.

20. Levy GA, and Marsden PA. Cigarette smoking—association with hepatic artery thrombosis. Liver Transplant 2002; 8(7): 588–590.

21. Pinna AD, Smith CV, Furukawa H, Starzl TE, and Fung JJ. Urgent revascularization of liver allografts after early hepatic artery thrombosis. Transplantation 1996; 62: 1584–1587.

22. Kusne S, and Blair JE. Viral and fungal infections after liver transplantation—part II Liver Transplant 2006; 12(1): 2–11.

23. Trauner M, Fickert P, and Stauber RE. Inflammation-induced cholestasis J Gastroenterol Hepatol 1999; 14(10): 946–959.

24. Lefkowitch JH. Bile ductular cholestasis: an ominous histopathologic sign related to sepsis and "cholangitis lenta" Hum Pathol 1982; 13(1): 19–24.

25. Paya CV, Hermans PE, Wiesner RH, et al. Cytomegalovirus hepatitis in liver transplantation: prospective analysis of 93 consecutive orthotopic liver transplantations J Infect Dis 1989; 160(5): 752–758.

26. Martelius T, Krogerus L, Hockerstedt K, Bruggeman C, and Lautenschlager I. Cytomegalovirus infection is associated with increased inflammation and severe bile duct damage in rat liver allografts. Hepatology 1998; 27(4): 996–1002.

27. Evans PC, Coleman N, Wreghitt TG, Wight DG, and Alexander GJ. Cytomegalovirus infection of bile duct epithelial cells, hepatic artery and portal

venous endothelium in relation to chronic rejection of liver grafts. J Hepatol 1999; 31(5): 913–920.

28. Lautenschlager I, Hockerstedt K, and Taskinen E. Histologic findings associated with CMV infection in liver transplantation. Transplant Proc 2003; 35(2): 819.

29. Lautenschlager I, Lappalainen M, Linnavuori K, Suni J, and Hockerstedt K CMV infection is usually associated with concurrent HHV-6 and HHV-7 antigenemia in liver transplant patients J Clin Virol 2002; 25(Suppl 2): S57–S61.

30. Chan FK, and Shaffer EA. Cholestatic effects of cyclosporine in the rat. Transplantation 1997; 63(11): 1574–1578.

31. Deters M, Klabunde T, Kirchner G, Resch K, and Kaever V. Sirolimus/ cyclosporine/tacrolimus interactions on bile flow and biliary excretion of immuno-suppressants in a subchronic bile fistula rat model. Br J Pharmacol 2002; 136(4): 604–612.

32. Sanchez-Campos S, Lopez-Acebo R, Gonzalez P, et al. Cholestasis and alterations of glutathione metabolism induced by tacrolimus (FK506) in the rat. Transplantation 1998; 66(1): 84–88.

33. Deters M, Kirchner G, Koal T, Resch K, and Kaever V. Everolimus/cyclosporine interactions on bile flow and biliary excretion of bile salts and cholesterol in rats. Dig Dis Sci 2004; 49(1): 30–37.

34. Romagnuolo J, Sadowski DC, Lalor E, Jewell L, and Thomson AB. Cholestatic hepatocellular injury with azathioprine: a case report and review of the mechanisms of hepatotoxicity. Can J Gastroenterol 1998; 12(7): 479–483.

35. Vierling JM, and Fennell RH. Jr. Histopathology of early and late human hepatic allograft rejection: evidence of progressive destruction of interlobular bile ducts Hepatology 1985; 5(6): 1076–1082.

36. Nawaz S, and Fennell RH. Apoptosis of bile duct epithelial cells in hepatic allograft rejection. Histopathology 1994; 25(2): 137–142.

37. Savier E, Lemasters JJ, and Thurman RG. Kupffer cells participate in rejection following liver transplantation in the rat. Transplant Int 1994; 7(Suppl 1): S183–S186.

38. Neuberger J. Incidence, timing, and risk factors for acute and chronic rejection. Liver Transplant Surg 1999; 5(4 Suppl 1): S30–S36.

39. Batts KP. Acute and chronic hepatic allograft rejection: pathology and classification. Liver Transplant Surg 1999; 5(4 Suppl 1): S21–S29.

40. Demetris AJ, Murase N, Ye Q, et al. Analysis of chronic rejection and obliterative arteriopathy. Possible contributions of donor antigen-presenting cells and lymphatic disruption. Am J Pathol 1997; 150(2): 563–578.

41. Neuberger J. Recurrent primary biliary cirrhosis. Liver Transplant 2003; 9(6): 539–546.

42. Sylvestre PB, Batts KP, Burgart LJ, Poterucha JJ, and Wiesner RH. Recurrence of primary biliary cirrhosis after liver transplantation: histologic estimate of incidence and natural history. Liver Transplant 2003; 9(10): 1086–1093.

43. Jacob DA, Neumann UP, Bahra M, Langrehr JM, and Neuhaus P. Liver transplantation for primary biliary cirrhosis: influence of primary immunosuppression on survival. Transplant Proc 2005; 37(4): 1691–1692.

44. Graziadei IW, Wiesner RH, Marotta PJ, et al. Long-term results of patients undergoing liver transplantation for primary sclerosing cholangitis. Hepatology 1999; 30(5): 1121–1127.

45. Goss JA, Shackleton CR, Farmer DG, et al. Orthotopic liver transplantation for primary sclerosing cholangitis. A 12-year single center experience. Ann Surg 1997; 225(5): 472–481.

46. Brandsaeter B, Schrumpf E, Bentdal O, et al. Recurrent primary sclerosing cholangitis after liver transplantation: a magnetic resonance cholangiography study with analyses of predictive factors. Liver Transplant 2005; 11(11): 1361–1369.

47. Kugelmas M, Spiegelman P, Osgood MJ, et al. Different immunosuppressive regimens and recurrence of primary sclerosing cholangitis after liver transplantation. Liver Transplant 2003; 9(7): 727–732.

48. Burak K, Angulo P, Pasha TM, et al. Incidence and risk factors for cholangiocarcinoma in primary sclerosing cholangitis. Am J Gastroenterol 2004; 99(3): 523–526.

49. Taga SA, Washington MK, Terrault N, et al. Cholestatic hepatitis C in liver allografts. Liver Transplant Surg 1998; 4(4): 304–310.

50. Cotler SJ, Taylor SL, Gretch DR, et al. Hyperbilirubinemia and cholestatic liver injury in hepatitis C-infected liver transplant recipients. Am J Gastroenterol 2000; 95(3): 753–759.

Index

183

Printed in the United States of America.